Ethical Issues in Nursing

This book examines major ethical issues in nursing practice. It eschews the abstract approaches of bioethics and medical ethics, and takes as its point of departure the difficulties nurses experience practising within the confines of a biomedical model and a hierarchical health care system. It breaks out of the rigid categories of mainstream health care ethics (autonomy, beneficence, quality of life, utilitarianism . . .) and provides case studies, experiences and challenging lines of thought for the new professional nurse.

The contributors examine the role of the nurse in relation to themes such as informed consent, privacy and dignity, and confidentiality. Nursing accountability is also considered in relation to the contemporary Western health care system as a whole. New and critical essays examine the nature of professional codes, care, medical judgement, nursing research and the law. Controversial issues, such as feeding those who cannot or will not eat, the epidemiology of HIV and dilemmas of choice and risk in the care of the elderly are tackled honestly and openly.

Geoffrey Hunt is the first philosopher to have been employed by the National Health Service. In 1992, his controversial National Centre for Nursing Ethics at the Hammersmith Hospital was closed down, reopening in 1993 at the University of East London. He has published widely in social philosophy and the ethics of health care.

Professional Ethics

General editors: Andrew Belsey and Ruth Chadwick
Centre for Applied Ethics, University of Wales College of Cardiff

Professionalism is a subject of interest to academics, the general public and would-be professional groups. Traditional ideas of professions and professional conduct have been challenged by recent social, political and technological changes. One result has been the development for almost every profession of an ethical code of conduct which attempts to formalise its values and standards. These codes of conduct raise a number of questions about the status of a 'profession' and the consequent moral implications for behaviour.

This series, edited from the Centre for Applied Ethics in Cardiff, seeks to examine these questions both critically and constructively. Individual volumes will consider issues relevant to particular professions, including nursing, genetic counselling, journalism, business, the food industry and law. Other volumes will address issues relevant to all professional groups such as the function and value of a code of ethics and the demands of confidentiality.

Also available in this series:

Ethical Issues in Journalism and the Media
Edited by Andrew Belsey and Ruth Chadwick

Ethical Issues in Social Work
Edited by Richard Hugman and David Smith

Genetic Counselling
Edited by Angus Clarke

The Ground of Professional Ethics
Daryl Koehn

Ethical Issues in Nursing

Edited by
Geoffrey Hunt

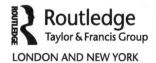

Routledge
Taylor & Francis Group

LONDON AND NEW YORK

First published 1994
by Routledge
Published 2014 by Routledge

2 Park Square, Milton Park, Abingdon, Oxon OX14 4RN
605 Third Avenue, New York, NY 10017, USA

Routledge is an imprint of the Taylor & Francis Group, an informa business

Introductory and editorial material © 1994 Geoffrey Hunt;
individual chapters © 1994 individual contributors; this
collection © 1994 Routledge

Typeset in Times Roman by
Computerset, Harmondsworth, Middlesex

British Library Cataloguing in Publication Data
A catalogue record for this book is available from the British
Library.

Library of Congress Cataloguing in Publication Data
Ethical Issues in Nursing / edited by Geoffrey Hunt.
p. cm. – (Professional ethics)
Includes bibliographical references and index.
1. Nursing ethics. I. Hunt, Geoffrey II. Series.
[DNLM: 1. Ethics, Nursing. WY 85 E838 1994]
RT85.E82 1994
174'.2–dc20 93-34921

ISBN 978-0-415-08144-3 (hbk)

Contents

Part II: General issues

Series editors' foreword

Applied Ethics is now acknowledged as a field of study in its own right. Much of its recent development has resulted from rethinking traditional medical ethics in the light of new moral problems arising out of advances in medical science and technology. Applied philosophers, ethicists and lawyers have devoted considerable energy to exploring the dilemmas emerging from modern health care practices and their effects on the practitioner–patient relationship.

But the point can be generalised. Even in health care, ethical dilemmas are not confined to medical practitioners but also arise in the practice of, for example, nursing. Studies of ethical issues in nursing, such as those contained in this book, have a vital role to play as nurse education and nursing practice change in parallel to new conceptions of health care delivery. Beyond health care, other groups are beginning to think critically about the kind of service they offer and about the nature of the relationship between provider and recipient. In many areas of life, social, political and technological changes have challenged traditional ideas of practice.

One visible sign of these developments has been the proliferation of codes of ethics, or of professional conduct. The drafting of such a code provides an opportunity for professionals to examine the nature and goals of their work, and offers information to others about what can be expected from them. If a code has a disciplinary function, it may even offer protection to members of the public.

But is the existence of such a code itself a criterion of a profession? What exactly is a profession? Can a group acquire professional status, and if so, how? Does the label 'professional' have implications, from a moral point of view, for acceptable behaviour, and if so how far do they extend?

This series, edited from the Centre for Applied Ethics in Cardiff and the Centre for Professional Ethics in Preston, seeks to examine these questions both critically and constructively. Individual volumes will address issues relevant to all professional groups, such as the nature of a profession, the function and value of codes of ethics, and the demands of confidentiality. Other volumes will examine issues relevant to particular professions, including those which have hitherto received little attention, such as journalism, social work and genetic counselling.

Andrew Belsey
Ruth Chadwick

Notes on contributors

Maddie Blackburn is Research Health Visitor in the Community Paediatric Research Unit, Chelsea and Westminster Hospital, London.

Donna Dickenson lectures in the Department of Health and Social Welfare at the Open University, Milton Keynes. She is the author of *Moral Luck in Medical Ethics and Practical Politics*, Avebury, 1991.

Andrew Edgar lectures in philosophy at the University of Wales College of Cardiff and is a member of the Centre for Applied Ethics at the university.

Julie Fenton is a Senior Dietitian, employed by Richmond, Twickenham and Roehampton Health Authority and working with people with learning difficulties. At the time she wrote her chapter she was working within the Mental Health Unit, Wandsworth Health Authority, London.

Linda Hanford is Head of the Department of Health Studies at the University of East London, London and Deputy Director of the European Centre for Professional Ethics.

Geoffrey Hunt is Director of the European Centre for Professional Ethics at the Institute of Health and Rehabilitation, University of East London, London. He has previously lectured in philosophy at the Universities of Swansea, Cardiff, Ife (Nigeria) and Lesotho.

Ann Kennedy is presently pursuing full-time doctoral studies at the London School of Hygiene and Tropical Medicine, University of London. She was previously Senior Research Nurse at St Mary's Hospital, Paddington, London.

Anne Maclean lectures in philosophy at the University College of Swansea. She previously lectured in philosophy at Newcastle University and Queen's University, Belfast. She is the author of *The Elimination of Morality*, published by Routledge.

Linda Smith is a Lecturer-Practitioner in Nursing, based at the Hammersmith Hospital and is a specialist in care of the elderly and in nursing research.

Deborah Taplin is Lecturer-Practitioner in Nursing, based at the Hammersmith Hospital and is a specialist in critical care.

Paul Wainwright is Programme Manager (Graduate Studies) for the Mid and West Wales College of Nursing & Midwifery, University College of Swansea. Before that he was a professional officer with the Welsh National Board for Nursing, Midwifery and Health Visiting, in Cardiff.

Ann P. Young is Deputy Registrar, The Nightingale and Guy's College of Nursing and Midwifery, Guy's Hospital, London and the author of several books on legal aspects of nursing.

Acknowledgements

I am especially grateful to nurse educators and nurses at the Hammersmith Hospital, London for warmly welcoming me, a social philosopher, into the National Health Service environment. As the first, and possibly the last, philosopher employed by the National Health Service I am lucky that I was allowed to be a gadfly for as long as two years. The University of East London had sufficient foresight to make it possible for me to continue my work.

Some formal acknowledgements are due. Julie Fenton's article arose in part from participation in the Royal College of Nursing's Nutrition Consensus Conference in November 1991. The views expressed in this article should not be taken to be representative of those of the Royal College of Nursing (RCN) or its Working Party on Nutritional Standards for the Older Adult. Thanks go to the Association for Spina Bifida and Hydrocephalus, for allowing the use of some of Maddie Blackburn's research materials in her chapter. I am grateful to the *Nursing Standard* for permission to use sections from my three articles on accountability: 'Professional Accountability', 1991, vol. 6 (4), pp. 49–50; 'Upward Accountability', 1992, vol. 6 (16), pp. 46–7; 'Downward Accountability', 1992, vol. 6 (21), pp. 44–5.

Bob Carley and Yvonne Bastin gave me help with alacrity in the nursing library at the Hammersmith Hospital. I thank Dr Ruth Chadwick and Mr Andrew Belsey of the University of Wales College of Cardiff for inviting me to edit this volume in their series.

I extend my warm appreciation to my friends Chris Stephens, Mike Cohen, Anne Maclean, and Colwyn Williamson for sharing times which were sometimes arduous, sometimes hilarious, but always very much alive.

Geoffrey Hunt

Introduction

Ethics, nursing and the metaphysics of procedure

Geoffrey Hunt

A PERENNIAL PREDICAMENT

On the whole the chapters in this volume adopt a standpoint which is rather different from the abstract rationalising standpoint of bioethics. More to the point, their approach is also somewhat different from that of mainstream medical ethics.

Throughout the chapters there appears some manifestation of that tortured predicament which has characterised nursing throughout its history. This predicament is either openly acknowledged and informs the thrust of the essay or it resides in underlying assumptions which give rise to certain unresolved difficulties and inadequacies. If I may put the predicament of nursing in overstated form for the sake of clarity: people, usually women, are given the special role of *caring* for other people on condition that they do so only under general direction from experts in the workings of the bodies of *Homo sapiens* and organised by experts in the management and administration of the mass treatment of these bodies. The perennial question posed is whether such means are adequate to the professed end. Is caring (not 'treatment', not 'curing' but *caring*) possible under such conditions? Is it possible only with great difficulty, heroic effort and exceptional people? The question perhaps is not whether it is *possible*, for the common decency and sometimes the heroic effort of individual nurses make it possible on a daily basis. The possibility is realised *despite* the health care system, not because of it. The proper question then is whether such a conception and such an arrangement facilitate caring or constantly work against it?

Naturally, the reality of nursing is far from being simple. The predicament is not always acutely felt and takes various forms. Many different activities, in many different kinds of setting, go under the name of nursing. Some nurses work in the community and others in research hospitals, some work with people who are well – trying to prevent illness – and others work with people who are critically ill but may make a full recovery, while yet others care for people who must shortly die. Some still work on large 'Nightingale wards' while others work in a small nursing home or hospice, and some work in large and constantly changing teams while others work in a 'primary nursing' manner. Some nurses work under great difficulties caused by an inflexible and hostile administrative regime or shortage of resources or both, while others are much luckier.

But through it all, I think, a general picture does emerge. In the hundreds of classroom and workplace discussions I have had with nurses, formally and informally, I have learned to distinguish between what is recurrent and systemic, and what may be put aside as peculiar, untypical or secondary.

Nurses often express unease about a lack of freedom to care for patients and clients as they feel is decent, as they feel they themselves would like to be cared for or have their loved ones cared for. Many, but not all, of the ethical issues they raise come back to this unease in one way or another. More often than not discussions end up in an exploration of the constraints on their freedom to care. Two general and related constraints, nearly always emerge: the way in which medicine defines health and illness, reflected in the way doctors think about and 'approach' people in care (the 'biomedical model'); and the way in which the whole business of health care, including nursing, is organised in a military-style command structure in which technical experts have the power (hierarchical technocracy). I am not suggesting any unanimity about this. Some nurses, usually the more senior ones disagree with me. They insist that there is nothing wrong as long as 'the professions' (medicine, management, nursing, etc.) 'respect' one another and work together in a 'team'. I suspect that in truth co-operation is limited and is for ever undermined by these deeper tensions and inconsistencies.

PROCEDURE

At a deeper level a source of a wide range of difficulties is the domination of nursing by a metaphysics of procedure, as is typical of administrative work in the civil service. Although it is true that individual nurses are highly respected, some are quite powerful, some are listened to carefully by doctors (especially junior doctors) and some care settings have good multidisciplinary policies, there is a strong general trend in nursing as a whole to keep an exaggerated quartermasterly discipline which runs counter to humane care. Every problem is conceived in terms of an appropriate procedure or sub-procedure or sub-sub-procedure. Procedure takes the form of uncritical habit and routine, excessive paper work and meetings, and unnecessary 'tests', 'obs' and 'monitoring'. Often it is tempting to slip into the rather dismal view that the nurse is simply there to follow instructions unquestioningly; just as the soldier is not expected to ask why he has to clean boots which are not dirty – in fact he is expected not to ask.

Time and effort is taken up with the constant search for the correct procedure; procedures are frequently checked and assessed to see that they are 'correct'; students are for the most part still taught by *reducing* every aspect of nursing to a procedure, so that even having a chat with a patient becomes a special procedure of 'communication' for which there is a science and a technique.

Taplin's small scale study (chapter 1) suggests that in at least one major London hospital (and there is no reason to suppose it to be untypical) informed consent is regarded as a procedure, very much like taking a temperature. Many nurses appear to think consent is principally about obtaining a signature (some wrongly think a relative's signature, or even a cross will do). Taplin emphasises that consent is not an administrative procedure but the moral demand to treat people in care with respect, making sure they understand and agree to what is being done to them.

Smith's research into falling accidents in the ward (chapter 3) also confirms the presence of rigid attitudes among nurses. Her study revealed that nurses made little attempt to understand the causes of falls, but were 'meticulous in merely reporting the falls' (p. 58-60). Blind adherence to procedure can be fatal, as the story of Mary illustrates. Furthermore, it is a short step from the observance of procedure to the habits of convenience: 'It is less trouble to wash an incontinent patient than take them to the lavatory regularly', says Smith (p. 67). Of course, the problem may be compounded by, and often originates in, a shortage of staff and resources.

I do not wish to say that there is no room for procedures or principles whatsoever in nursing practice. Having said that, however, I still feel that many procedures and principles which are necessary are *made* necessary by the defects which arise from the general organisation and ideology of health care. Thus one would like to see better procedures for maintaining accountability to people in care and ensuring that nurses are allowed a voice, but this is only necessary because the organisational culture of health care needs democratic renewal as a whole. To give another example, Wainwright (chapter 2) presents a set of principles for maintaining the privacy and self-respect of people in care, and these are to be welcomed (p. 52-53). But the question remains why it should be necessary to state such principles at all. I would say that new procedures are welcome in so far as they have an educative role in bringing about cultural renewal, a renewal which would ultimately take away the emphasis on obedience to procedure.

'MORAL TECHNOLOGY' OR ETHICAL EXPLORATION?

Ethics is being added to the nursing curriculum up and down the land: an hour on anatomy, an hour on physiology, an hour on ethics, an hour on wound management, an hour on pressure sores, and so on. What purpose does this serve? What difference does or can it make? Will it change the way nurses think about their work? Will it change it fundamentally? Will it improve nursing, making it more decent, more humane?

Many ethics courses presuppose that nurses have a need for 'help with moral decision making' and that to satisfy this need they should be taught 'moral concepts' or 'principles' or even 'moral theory'. It is assumed that nurses need yet another *procedure*, a framework of rules, which they can apply to the situations they encounter at work.

It is curious how in many ways a lot of nursing ethics now taking shape on curricula imitates the technocratic and curative approach to health. As is generally recognised (often in the same documents which make a case for nursing ethics), instead of looking for and dealing with the conditions which give rise to illness, our health care system invites us to bombard the victim with the latest scientific wonder – radiation, chemicals, lasers, ultrasound, gene-carrying viruses or what you will – and very often makes matters worse. In the case of ethics many appear convinced that a heavy dose of theories and principles carrying labels like 'deontology or utilitarianism', 'beneficence', 'non-maleficence', 'autonomy', 'quality or sanctity of life' will fill the moral void in our health care system.

Yet surely everyone knows that student nurses do *already* have the responses of honesty, promise-keeping, respect for others, privacy, self-esteem and do understand these concepts. There is no reason to suppose teachers to be morally superior to students. The problem does not lie in some sort of moral ignorance to be rectified with the latest in moral technology. Most people come to their health care workplace and put on their uniforms already equipped with everything human they need to treat the people in their care decently. The problem is that the circumstances and character of nursing do not allow them to do so. To shed one's mufti and don a uniform is to be required to shed one's moral sense and don the metaphysics of procedure.

In ethical discussion about nursing practice it is not easy to steer clear of the temptation to start off by describing and analysing 'moral concepts'. Wainwright mentions some attempts to define 'privacy' which in turn leads to attempts to define 'person' and so on (p. 43). One has to be careful to avoid any suggestion that the reason privacy is on the whole not well respected in health care institutions is that the health carers stand in need of a clear definition of 'privacy' or 'dignity' or 'person'.

All this is not to say that student nurses cannot benefit from moral debate about health care matters and situations, and learn from instruction in professional ethics and the law. I take it for granted that the debate is illuminating and the instruction useful.

What one has to beware of is making the problem appear to be one of finding the technically right procedure or method for dealing with 'ethical decisions', as though the problem were similar in kind to finding the right medication or the right diagnosis or the right administrative rule. This diverts attention away from an inquiry into the concrete realities which make decent care difficult or impossible. Far from making the situation better, this technical–ethical approach makes it worse.

Nurses need ethical exploration. That is, they need freely to examine from cases, preferably in their own experience, the conditions which create disparities between what their ordinary moral sense tells them and what they are expected to do without question, expected to accept, believe and justify without moral doubt or anxiety. Of course, it may be convenient to begin the discussion with a theme such as 'confidentiality' or 'consent', but not along the line of 'applying a principle' which in practice turns out to be irrelevant or even oppressive.

Readers looking into this volume for moral theory, or for reasoning from principles such as 'autonomy' or 'justice', will be disappointed. These studies are intended to prompt readers ethically to explore for themselves real situations and difficulties – that is the only strength I would hope this collection has.

WHOSE ETHICS

To work 'successfully' in the health care system, then, is to accept a metaphysics, and an ideology – to accept a way of working which has evolved over decades and is there waiting to receive one on its terms. If one does not accept those terms one is unlikely to be employed, and if one is employed then one may find oneself at best merely tolerated and at worst expelled. Nursing education has always been more than a training in anatomy, physiology and nursing tasks – it has been an ideological preparation, even an indoctrination. The fear is that nursing ethics, while hoping or pretending to break with the old, may be appropriated, may become part of that metaphysics of procedure.

Ethics has made its appearance on the nursing agenda because of a crisis of legitimation in the health care of the Western world. People are losing confidence in the orthodoxy. Health care technocracy has reached a state of development at which, despite its achievements, its failings are generally manifest and its promises exposed as hollow at the same time that its power has become unbearably overweening – this is especially evident in North America perhaps. Health care ethics is perhaps the system's promise to clean up its own act, and clean it up on its own terms. The danger is that the professional under threat by a disenchanted public will soon, armed with a Masters degree in Health Care Ethics, make claim to a new expertise – moral expertise. Yet another way of fielding questions from dissatisfied patients, clients and their families? I worry about this partly because the question of the public accountability of the health care management (as opposed to the accountability of individual nurses) is still unresolved and the ethics teachers and textbooks are strangely silent on this wider issue. One may suspect that 'ethics' began where public accountability failed. The danger is that a democratic deficit is being filled with philosophical jargon. To put it differently, positive ethics, the ethics of theorising and expert moralising would, I believe, be dissolved by ubiquitous public accountability and public control. The question

'Whose ethics?' is fundamental. Who defines it as a 'field' in the first place, who controls it, who benefits from it? It is natural perhaps to suppose that 'ethics' is something standing outside all the real world conflicts in the health care arena – as something which experts (mostly utilitarian and rationalist philosophers) have special access to and can convey to the health care professional so that 'everyone will benefit'. The health carer learns some moral theory, learns to speak in a largely incomprehensible fashion ('universalisability', 'non-maleficence', 'consequentialist', 'intrinsic value', 'supererogatory', 'value of life') and is supposedly all the better for it, ready to apply her new-found ethics to the real world.

Still, things are not so bleak. One may instead *apply the real world to ethics*. Listening to people in care (for example, some of Taplin's interviewees or Smith's elderly people, in these pages) one may learn to approach ethics differently. The crisis of legitimation provides an opportunity for cultural renewal, for an ethics of resistance to stultifying biomedical bureaucracy. After all, is not the problem really one of the conditions and constraints of the health care institution in which people work, constraints which often engender fear, paralysis and at worst a kind of blindness necessary to preserve the integrity of the self? If so, this suggests the need for what may be called a *negative ethics*, an ethics which, instead of trying to tell people what is right, allows them to discuss what is wrong, to investigate what it is that does not allow them to do what is right or, sometimes, see what is right. This would be a critique of our health care practices by encouraging a self-discovery of the obstacles, of whatever kind, to acting in ways which we know to be right. I say this aware of the dangers of adopting some moral standpoint from which to indoctrinate students anew. I do not intend to promote any such standpoint, but rather to facilitate the emergence of various standpoints out of the honest and rigorous examination of issues posed by nurses and their teachers. Conflicts between the modes of thought of 'professionals' and so-called 'lay' people, of nurses and doctors, of management and employees in relation to health and health care need to be critically examined. Such a need is recognised at once by the neophyte nurse, if sometimes accepted with greater reluctance by the nurse who has practised for many years and has come to accept the norms of the institution. To undertake this kind of negative and exploratory ethics requires the opportunity and the freedom openly to tease out the inconsistencies in thinking about the nature of nursing and to seek their origin, to discuss the history and politics of nursing, its place in contemporary life and its relation to major social issues such as the environment and civil rights.

MODES OF THOUGHT

The root of the problems of modern health care, and modern nursing, may well be perceived as one of increasing demands, rising costs and dwindling revenue or as inefficient management and administration. The root may equally and perhaps more fruitfully be perceived as a problem of conception, of our contemporary mode of thinking about illness, health and health care.

The viability of a biomedical and technocratic health care system depends on a certain kind of perception of people who have certain setbacks in life. People have first to be identified as 'patients', and these people have also to go along most of the time with such an identification. The patient is an *object* of medical science (human biology and pathology), a science which cannot be separated from the organisational form it takes. Thus it transpires from these chapters, as I have mentioned, that one general obstacle to decent care is indeed the concept of 'patient' itself, the dysfunctional specimen of *Homo sapiens* receiving expert biological intervention. The other closely related general obstacle flows from the characteristics of the organisation – the 'nurse' as obedient technical assistant, as a subordinate element in a command structure. The health care system, despite recent changes, still has an almost military-industrial configuration.

Thus, to restate, the most radical ethical question for nursing is this: is obedience to procedures designed for the mass treatment of dysfunctional organisms adequate to the task of caring for people who need help with setbacks of a particular kind? This creates a novel and wide agenda for nursing ethics, one which gets away from the endless repetition of 'principles' and abstract theories. What kinds of setbacks are indeed 'health' setbacks? What kinds of professional and personal attitudes are engendered in those who perceive people as dysfunctional organisms? What is a 'professional' and what are the kinds and limits of professional knowledge? What are the connections between knowledge and power? Do nurses have to be obedient and disciplined, and if so in what ways and why? Why is the accountability of nurses emphasised but the accountability of health authorities and hospital management hardly ever raised?

BIOMEDICAL MODEL

Such questions go beyond the notion of ethics as dealing with proper conduct, with malpractice and negligence. Here is an ethical endeavour which challenges *standard* practice, which recognises that, even where everything is in accordance with set rules and procedures and no one can be blamed for any wrongdoing, still something may be radically wrong. Honesty, for example, is an ethical imperative which goes far beyond matters such as the wrongness of stealing patients' property or drugs from the medicines' cabinet. Those questions of professional honesty (which are not without their importance, of course) leave quite untouched the deeper issue of whether our perceptions, justifications and reasoning about illness and disease and our remedies for them are dishonest, an illusion serving narrow interests. Thus the obstetrician may be perfectly honest and conduct himself 'ethically' as a professional in emphasising 'risks' and 'abnormality' and bring the expectant mother under his control where she may be 'monitored'. But what if this control is unnecessary? What if, as evidence strongly suggests, home births are safer than hospital births? What if monitoring has unacknowledged dangers? What if the mother finds the hospital delivery upsetting or even humiliating? The ethical question then moves to a deeper level – is it a misconception that contemporary obstetric care is good and right?

To take some other examples from this volume. Smith's contribution (chapter 3) challenges the assumption that the old are dependent and burdensome. Her chapter suggests to me that contemporary health care arrangements require and even create dependence. Elderly people are perhaps perfect objects for such a system. While economic arrangements continue to make the elderly people dependent and promote a perception of 'the old' and even 'the geriatric', health care completes the picture by building its own power on the dependence so created. Certainly Smith poses a genuine dilemma of dependence or risk. However, it is all too easy to slip into the assumption that the needs of the health care system are the proper measure of the care of old people. If it is asked, apparently as an ethical question, how far can elderly people in care be allowed to make choices, are we really asking the question of how far we professionals can *allow* patients to make those choices which will be burdensome to us, creating more work, more legal liabilities, and so on? It is unlikely that a person in care would regard this as an ethical (moral) question.

Wainwright mentions situations in which people in care suffer various indignities and invasions of privacy (p. 50). The biomedical perception of, and attitude towards, people in care is bound to a general tendency to alienate and demean. Nurses have participated in this alienation to a large degree. Why were routine enemas once thought necessary? And why are they now thought unnecessary? – Probably because they were discovered to be clinically irrelevant rather than because it was realised that they were an offence to the patient. Consider the woman admitted to the labour ward, flat on her back with her legs up in stirrups, students and other strangers moving around her, often more attention being given to the monitors than to her. She may well feel alienated, an object for obstetric procedures. Fortunately, this is changing, and changing largely under the impact of resistance from mothers and midwives. Still, Wainwright is right to draw attention to the way in which nurses stand in constant danger of being 'desensitised' in an environment in which care is understood as a technical enterprise.

Fenton, who is a dietitian, also highlights some ethical repercussions of biomedical health care in chapter 4. Many ethical problems of feeding did not arise before modern technology came along. And of course it is not as though modern technology, as a collection of machines and operating instructions, can easily be separated from a way of thinking in terms of machines, a machine-like way of thinking. The recovery of nursing care requires not so much more thinking about the 'proper place of technology', but rather less technological thinking. Feeding has always been a part of nursing care, but of late it has become more of a technical process and a part of medical treatment.

Fenton makes clear that the presence of a nasogastric tube is not just a matter of some discomfort (which would define the ethical issue as one of making the patient as comfortable as possible, etc.) but of self-esteem. There is a loss of control and choice about food; the person in care may perceive herself as the appendage of a machine.

DOCTORS AND NURSES

Fenton's contribution, like many of the others, raises issues about the nursing role and its relation to medicine. Feeding, by new means, may be acceptable as a supportive measure while the patient recovers from some illness. But what if the prospect of recovery is slim and the patient tells the nurses he does not want artificial feeding? Feeding may prolong suffering. In other situations the doctors may wish to terminate artificial feeding, and the nurses may feel very reluctant to go along with this. More or less coherent differences in the perceptions and approaches, and indeed the attitudes, of doctors and nurses appear to lie behind such disagreements. (Sometimes, of course, in any *particular* disagreement one could not say, if one did not see the uniforms, which were the views of the nurses and which of the doctors.) If feeding is a 'medical intervention' then the nurse may be pushed out of an area that traditionally was hers.

The case of an elderly patient called Arthur, which is raised by Smith (pp. 62-4), is illuminating in this regard. Arthur pleaded for a cessation of treatment and the nurses took his part although the doctors insisted on continuing. In the event Arthur recovered. Smith appears to doubt, rightly I think, that a mistake had been made by the nurses (and the patient and relatives). Was it a mistake? The point is that the medical staff refused even to consider stopping treatment. If their action was not a *considered* one, reached through sensitive discussion with patient, relatives and nurses, how could they regard themselves as 'right' simply because the treatment worked? One may be justified in suspecting that there is a dogma or a fear at work here – the dogma that if the body usually responds well to treatment then it is always right to treat the patient; the fear that litigation might follow if one does not strive officiously to keep the patient alive. If Arthur had died when he might have lived does it follow that the carers would have been wrong, under the circumstances, to withhold treatment? Would we not be justified in pointing out, among other things, that that was a risk *he* was perfectly prepared to take?

Another aspect of the case of Arthur is this: the doctors may smugly say 'we were right' thereby undermining the confidence of nurses and making them feel inferior – as though their judgement was (and usually is) inferior. But was their judgement inferior? Was it not rather that different considerations went into their judgement; it was a different kind of judgement – perhaps a more immediate, personal and caring one. We may ask this question: if it had gone the other way and Arthur had died a prolonged and miserable death under the treatment regime, would the doctors come forward and say 'Oh, sorry, we got it wrong'? They might, or we might expect them to say, 'We did our best, as we were obliged to do.' But would this have been their best? And what sense of best? *Clinical* best? Moral best?

Tensions between medicine and nursing are increasingly coming to the fore in the field of health care research. In the past, says Blackburn in chapter 5, 'Many nurses merely assumed the role of data collectors for doctors and medical researchers without necessarily questioning their actions or responsibilities' (p. 103). Blackburn, a research health visitor, looks at the responsibilities of the nurse researcher. She refers to her research into the sexuality of adolescents with spina bifida and hydrocephalus. Doctors tend to conceptualise health care practice in dualistic fashion – the technical on one hand and the moral/ethical on the other. The former is taken to be their special preserve, while ethics committees and lawyers look after the latter. Blackburn says at the beginning of her chapter that ethical considerations are 'as integral and important as the research "methods" and "results"' (p. 90). An example of an obvious way in which a concern strictly with 'science' and 'technique' is untenable is provided by Blackburn's discovery in the course of her research that some of the adolescents had been abused. Should she ignore this, sticking only to what 'science' requires?

Although this researcher's work was non-therapeutic, it was always envisaged as having fairly direct benefits for the disabled in general. Other non-therapeutic research, which nurses may be involved in as 'assistants', may not clearly have any benefits at all. What is the nursing standpoint on this fact? If we uncritically accept strict professional boundaries the answer may be easy – nurses have no standpoint. But do we accept? In fact, a general question about the structure of health care is how far professional boundaries prevent ethical issues being identified or raised or resolved, and indeed how far the boundaries even define and create them in the first place. Thus one comes across situations in which apparently doctors are absolved from ethical worries by a strict concern with science and technique, nurses absolved by a subordinate preoccupation with executing procedure, managers absolved by a concern with money and efficiency, politicians by a concern with the econ-

omy, and the public and patients are disempowered. Responsibility
has no place to reside. Meanwhile, health care practice is subdivided
into dozens of specialisms (cardiology, theatre nursing, midwifery,
occupational therapy, dietetics and podiatry, etc.), a subdivision
which diffuses responsibility and leads to scapegoating and buck-
passing. Blackburn notes that, 'Unfortunately, it happens too frequently that the people who provide the research data are the last to
have access to it, to read it, and to benefit from it.'

An area of research in which nurses have had little voice is that of
HIV/AIDS epidemiology. Kennedy's essay (chapter 6) brings specifically nursing concerns to her experience of working in this field for
some years, where she never lost sight of the person at the end of the
technocratic chain. Kennedy writes, 'the conflicts and power struggles which still exist between medicine and nursing make it very
difficult for nurses – advocates of their patients – to live by the letter
and spirit of their code' (p. 107).

Kennedy illustrates the concerns of the nurse through the story of
Amanda who, together with her baby, is HIV positive and unexpectedly finds herself subjected to an interview by an epidemiologist-
researcher who has traced her through a general practitioner's
record, a record which should have been treated in confidence.
What makes matters worse is that Amanda had been tested for HIV
without her knowledge and therefore without her consent and the
researcher had not submitted his research proposal to a research
ethics committee for approval in the first place. This was non-
therapeutic research and was not intended to benefit Amanda or
any other individual.

Taking 'patient advocacy' seriously, Kennedy sees nurses assuming an ethical lead and doing so corporately. Nurses should be
applying pressure for the reform of ethical review in the UK. It is
unsatisfactory that such review is still medically dominated, nurses
being grossly under-represented.

Maclean (chapter 11) gets closer to the conceptual root of the
problem which has been raised here. She is concerned with the
concept of 'medical judgement' ('clinical judgement'). She makes
her point by examining a text written by a doctor. Active voluntary
euthanasia is said to be a moral judgement and not a medical
judgement, and therefore no part of medicine. It is said, at the same
time, that withholding life-support may be a purely medical judgement – one can on a purely clinical basis determine what is in the
best interests of the patient. The right time to die can, supposedly,

be clinically determined in some cases. But Maclean takes issue with this, arguing that a closer examination of so-called medical judgements in question reveals them to be no different in kind from so-called moral judgements.

I would say that medical talk of the 'interest of the patient' is in the doctor's mind talk about the biological interest of the human body – which is where medical expertise lies. But there's an unsustainable dualism here. When the doctor talks of my body he talks of *me*. To make a decision about my body is to make a decision about me. Medical experts have to be careful not to act as moral experts under the mantle of medical judgement.

TECHNOCRACY

The question of obedience to the dictates of a biomedical technocratic system takes the guise of a renewed concern with 'accountability' in nursing. In my contribution (chapter 7) I ask, rather provocatively, whether ethical practice is possible in nursing. Nurses have little or no freedom, so accountability is perhaps only of a military character. What is the significance of so much recent talk about nursing accountability? Is it about adjustment to the new quasi-market in health care, an adjustment which is supposed to leave unasked questions about the accountability of the management of purchaser and provider units: health authorities, trusts, etc.? Nursing is defined and moulded and driven by forces outside nursing and which nursing has never really understood or challenged. How far is self-regulation and upward (line management) accountability able to serve the public good and thus serve the truth in nursing, the truth of nursing? The circle is broken, can it be closed, and how?

I am critical of an imposed discipline which nurses feel as an external force curtailing their freedom to act out of common decency and compassion. For too long nurses have been treated as though they cannot be trusted, as though they are infantile. Some managers and representatives of professional bodies speak disdainfully of the alternative as a kind of anarchy in which everyone appeals to his or her 'conscience', whatever it may be. It does not appear to occur to them that the conscience of nurses as nurses is, or can become, a social attribute – that is, it is what the individual feels in the very act of expressing a collective social responsibility. Responsibility need not be experienced as an external discipline, nor as mere subjective opinion, but as the solidarity of the group residing in the conscience of its members.

In chapter 8 Edgar pursues some of my points in relation to professional codes in particular. He explores the relation between a professional code of conduct, such as the United Kingdom Central Council's (UKCC) code for nurses, and the moral sense of ordinary (lay) people. After all, nurses are ordinary people with the moral attitudes and beliefs of society before they are professionals. While making sense of any code by professionals actually depends on the ordinary moral sense we must all have, a code also serves to regulate a profession (and a profession has some interests of its own) and tensions and conflicts may thus arise.

Making use of the concept of 'life world' (taken from thinkers such as Husserl, Schutz, and Habermas), Edgar opens up the question of the interpretation of any code – it is always more or less open, and conflicting readings are possible. Indeed, this possibility is necessary for the ideological function which codes have – to paper over differences of interest, allowing one reading when it suits the professional (an 'insulating' function), one when it suits manage-ment and another when it suits the public. Edgar notes (pp. 159–60) that the UKCC's code assumes nursing progress rests on the 'excel-lence of its individual practitioners'. But individualism, and ideas about excellence, themselves need re-examination together with a gamut of other concepts, some of which I have been mooting in this introduction. Young, in chapter 9, takes much more for granted than the pieces by Edgar and myself, but her essay still poses some important challenges in our understanding of the relation between law, workplace policies and professional ethics. Young says, 'Con-tractual obligations should mirror professional standards, and to some extent do' (p. 177); but not completely. When standards drop due to resource insufficiency then professional ethics demands caution or complaint, while contractual obligations demand that one carry on regardless. To report low standards of care may mean victimisation at work, while not to report them may leave the practitioner open to professional discipline. Young suggests that the nurses' code of conduct could be reinforced by linking it with the contract of employment. This would improve matters for nurses and patients. However, 'some employers are not ready to face the implications of raising the status of the Code in this way', she adds (p. 168). There are other conflicts. The UKCC's code requires that

nurses should ensure patients give informed consent and a supporting document states that nurses may even go as far as refusing to
participate if they are sure the patient does not understand; but to go
against doctors and managers may mean facing workplace discipline
for insubordination.

Certainly, as long as inconsistencies continue to exist between
the requirements of the workplace and of the profession then
whistleblowing, victimisation and big compensation pay-outs from
public money will continue.

CARE

Nearly everyone agrees that nursing is about care and, as we have
seen, many of the chapters raise questions about the constraints on
care. But does the concept of care itself need examination? An
examination which springs naturally from an exploration of nursing's difficulties need not be diversionary and could be fruitful.
But, as I have already suggested in the case of other moral concepts,
the idea that we must *first* get clear about the concept as a kind of
'first principle' could well be diversionary and fruitless. In my view,
many nurse theorists, mostly American, have adopted the latter
approach.

In chapter 10 Hanford examines Nel Noddings' theory of care
propounded in her 1984 book *Caring: A Feminine Approach to
Ethics and Moral Education*, although she has doubts: 'No doubt
one has to be somewhat suspicious of theories of morality, all of
which are reductionist in one way or another' (p. 196). Noddings'
book has been seminal in the United States, especially in the debate
about moral education, but has hardly entered into the debate about
nursing.

Noddings sees care as the true basis of ethical behaviour. If this is
true, since caring is said by many to be the essence of nursing,
Noddings' work might be expected to have something important to
say for nursing ethics. She distinguishes between natural caring and
ethical caring and maintains that the latter arises from the former.
Nursing has always faced what Hanford refers to as 'the difficulty of
caring for someone for whom we do not naturally care'. Noddings
appears to give us a clue as to how this works. One may not naturally
care for the patient x, or even wish to do so, but ethical caring still
depends on natural caring in so far as it is a recognition of what one
ought to feel, of getting a grip on one's better self, so to speak, in

encouraging oneself into a better attitude – a bit like cheering oneself up, or psyching oneself up for a long jump.

The reality of the circumstances in which nursing occurs is often so dire nowadays that it seems academic to consider such questions. But Noddings recognised that prior conditions must be met for ethical caring. Hanford speaks of nursing having to practise in a 'chronically ethically diminished state'. Nursing administration needs to create an environment, she suggests, where conditions for care may flourish.

In chapter 12 Dickenson also raises questions about care, examining nurse time treated as a resource. I think her case runs into great difficulties, pointing to a deeper question – does it make sense to treat as a 'resource' time spent caring? Dickenson takes her starting point from a debate in medical ethics, which perhaps explains her approach. A great deal of medical ethics is about the consideration of various criteria for allocating resources, for example, kidney transplants. The author thinks that clinical and social criteria are not plausible when we look at dividing the most valuable nursing resource – nurse time. Dickenson's principal question is: how does a nurse ethically divide up her time between patients?

Any nurse can see that an unsavable dying patient may need more care than others, not less. She thinks nurse autonomy and randomisation should be considered as alternative criteria. The first means that nurses should make up their own mind on a case basis. (I doubt that this is a criterion at all, and the reason it is not could be very enlightening if examined.) The second gets all her attention. Dickenson calls it randomisation. The idea is that once a nursing judgement has been made about time for the pressing cases, one should divide up the remainder equally. This way at least one would be treating people as equals, and ruling out personal bias. Dickenson seems a little shy about defending this idea without qualification, and probably with good reason, although I do not think this reason actually emerges. After all, she is only talking about 'residual time', and even then warns that 'There is no reason why she [the nurse] has to equalise her time mechanically' (p. 213).

What an examination of any 'ethical criteria for allocating resources' shows, I think, is that there is something misconceived here. (This is not the place to argue this out in full.) Our efforts should perhaps be aimed in quite different directions – for example, why there is scarcity at all and what can be done about it?

Perhaps the point is best made by a powerful story which Dickenson uses to make her case. I think this story can be turned around, against her case. A shipwreck survivor called Holmes was blamed by a judge for using social criteria (age, family relationship, etc.) for deciding who should be thrown off an overloaded lifeboat. The judge thought drawing straws (equalisation) was the only fair method. It is incidental in the story that two sisters had jumped overboard to drown with their brother, who had been jettisoned. The sisters' action is what is significant to me. It may look peculiar from the point of view of any method, but we should perhaps take the line that if the sisters' action is perfectly understandable, even heroic and moving, then it is the idea of a method (procedure) which is peculiar in this context.

There is a limit to what in health care lends itself to rational principle, procedure and method. Unfortunately, the success of contemporary biomedical and technocratic health care requires a failure to recognise and respect this limit.

Part I

Specific issues

Chapter 1

Nursing and informed consent
An empirical study

Deborah Taplin

In 1985 I had reason, as a nurse, to interview a 36-year-old woman who was about to undergo a hysterectomy. A glance at her medical history revealed that she had undergone a tubal ligation ten years earlier and was therefore sterile. In the interview she told me that the most upsetting aspect of the impending surgery was the fact that she would, as a result, be unable to have any more children. She was surprised to learn that she was already sterile. In this case the consent procedure had not been followed. I wondered how many more such cases there were in British hospitals.

In 1990 I undertook a pilot project at a major university hospital in London to investigate competent adult patients' understanding of the surgical treatment which they had received.[1] My hypothesis was that an adequate consent procedure was not being followed. Although the results may not be representative of every hospital ward in the UK, there is plenty of informal and anecdotal evidence to suggest that the situation I found is not untypical for many British hospitals. As the majority of the medical and nursing staff I came into contact with were, or will be, employed in other hospitals it is quite unlikely that the behaviour observed is unique to the particular setting studied.

Furthermore, a study by Byrne, Napier and Cuschieri carried out in a British surgical unit in 1987 showed that of a hundred patients interviewed twenty-seven did not know which organ was operated on and forty-four were unaware of the exact nature of the surgical process.[2]

I gave a structured interview to twenty men who had undergone a trans-urethral resection of the prostate and eighteen women who had had a dilatation and curettage. Granted the limitations and possible errors of a pilot study of this kind, the results still make dismal reading. On the whole, I found that inadequate pre-operative information had been given. If a signature was present on a consent form then patients and medical and nursing staff appeared satisfied. These findings supported my hypothesis.

CONSENT IN GENERAL

I briefly set out here some general points about consent, to set the scene. Many of these points appear in the Department of Health's recent guidelines, which every nurse should be familiar with.[3]

A patient has a right to withhold consent for examination or treatment, or withdraw it at any time. Consent is important in the law because of its connection with trespass to the person, that is, assault or battery. An assault is any act which causes in the person subjected to it an apprehension of the immediate infliction of a battery. A battery is the physical contact with another's person. To have obtained informed consent is a defence against an accusation of assault and/or battery.

Consent may be express, when it is oral or written down, and this is the usual practice for surgical procedures. It is implied, for example in compliant actions such as raising one's arm for an injection. Implied consent may be adequate for minor procedures.

The most important element in consent is the patient's under-standing of what is going to be done. Obtaining valid consent involves giving an explanation of the nature of the examination or treatment, of any substantial risks involved, of any side-effects and consequences for the life of the patient, mentioning alternatives, and giving all this information in a form which is comprehensible to the patient. Of course, the patient may be advised about a course of action, but it is important to back up this advice with the reasons.

In general one cannot give consent for another person. As Bridgit Dimond has explained: 'There is no authority in law, apart from that given to the parent of a minor under 18, where a relative can give a valid consent for a patient.'[4] As one might expect, there are circumstances where it would be right to give treatment without consent, such as for saving the life of an unconscious patient or to treat a mental disorder of a patient liable to be held in hospital under the Mental Health Act. I will be concerned here only with the consent of competent adults to surgical treatment in hospital.

THE RESEARCH STUDY

Method

I chose to use a structured interview rather than a self-completing questionnaire because I believe the interview is less likely to restrict the kinds of reply given. I was aware that I should not lead the patient's answer.

To be admitted as a subject on the study each patient had to be: a) at least 18 years of age, b) able to speak and understand English, and c) mentally competent. Having obtained ethical approval for the study, subjects were initially identified on operating lists, and once on the wards I relied on the assessment of a registered nurse to decide which patients would be asked to participate.

In total twenty-five men who had undergone a trans-urethral resection of the prostate (TURP) and twenty-five women who had had a dilatation and curettage (D & C) were approached. Twenty-two men agreed to take part. Two of these were not admissible, one because he was very deaf and appeared to be disoriented and the other because he did not speak English. Eighteen women agreed to participate. This gave me a group consisting of thirty-eight people in all.

All the interviews were conducted post-operatively. They took place any time from four hours after surgery for 'day patients' to the second or third day after surgery for in-patients. One subject had had two operations and his interview was conducted after the second one.

The interviews were designed to establish the patients' views about the consent procedure and to discover how much information each had been given as a basis for making an informed decision about treatment. Towards the end of 1989 the Department of Health issued 'A Guide to Consent for Examination or Treatment'; this circular supported my thinking and added weight to the study.

Only eight simple questions were asked. I was aware that it was important to make the questions non-threatening, understandable and easy to answer.

Results

I now present the results, question by question. I list the answers given with the numbers of patients giving that answer or one very like it. Answers that were essentially the same were grouped.

1 Why did you need an operation?

Men's answers: dribbling of urine 3; referred by GP for another health problem, enlarged prostate then noticed 1; emergency admission 3; failure of balloon dilatation 2; nocturea 4; enlarged prostate 2; referred by another specialist 1; problems for over six months 1; unable to pass urine and attempt to catheterise failed 2; haematurea 1.

Women's answers: menorrhagia and fibroids or post-birth erosion 2; menorrhagia 4; irregular bleeding and polyps or hormone problems 3; vaginal discharge 1; post-partum haemorrhage 1; period problems 1; did not want a hysterectomy 1; irregular bleeding 3; dysmenorrhoea and polyps/fibroids 2.

2 When did you find out you needed treatment?

Men's answers: outpatients' department one to four weeks ago 3; one to three months ago 6; three months to one year ago 1; one to four years ago 5; emergency admission 3; after admission 2.

Women's answers: outpatients' department (OPD) one to four weeks ago 8; one to three months ago 1; discussed with GP 3; OPD appointment and GP 1; OPD appointment 3; heard of endometrial ablation and sought information 1; told needed hysterectomy in OPD, told of D & C on admission 1.

One man had been waiting for treatment for one month at the study hospital, but longer at another hospital. Another who had been admitted as an emergency had been in hospital for several days before learning of the proposed operation. Of those who were waiting one to four years: one man's treatment had been delayed due to social problems and waiting list delays; one man had had some other treatment first; one man had another medical problem; and two of the men were having a second or fourth operation.

3 What operation did you have?

Men were given a choice of: a) Prostatectomy, b) TURP, and c) trans-urethral resection of the prostate. Women were given a choice of: a) dilatation and curettage and b) D & C. (It transpired during the interviews that only three women had D & C only on the consent form; the remaining women had had another procedure as well, such as laparoscopy or hysteroscopy. This is a design fault in the study.) The subjects were asked to identify either from memory or from the list which operation they had had. Most of the women had also undergone another medical procedure and they were also asked to identify that. I compared the replies given with the relevant written consent forms to see if the answers were the same.

Operation on the men's consent form: TURP 9; TURP and cystoscopy 3; TURP and retrograde ejaculation 3; trans-urethral resection of the prostate 2; TURP and trans-urethral resection of the prostate 1; TURP and orchidectomy 1; bladder neck incision 1.

An additional consent form for a man who had had a haemorrhage after his TURP and needed vaginal packs inserted into the prostate bed, showed 'removal of vaginal packs'.

Operation described by men: Did not know 13; possibly a trans-urethral resection of prostate 1; did not remember 1; prostatectomy 3; unsure, perhaps a prostatectomy 2.

Of the thirteen who said they did not know, one did not appear to understand what the operation was, judging by his description of the procedure. The man who had had the reactionary bleeding necessitating a second operation did not know what operation he had undergone on either occasion.

Operation on the women's consent form: D & C and hysteroscopy 12; D & C and polypectomy 1; D & C 2; D & C, hysteroscopy and polypectomy 1; laparoscopic sterilisation 1; tubal ligation, removal of intra-uterine contraceptive device (IUCD), D & C and hysteroscopy 1.

Comparing the men's consent forms with their statements we find that of those who were partially correct, one stated he had had a trans-urethral resection of the prostate and had signed his consent form for a TURP and retrograde ejaculation. One was unsure but thought he had had a prostatectomy, although his consent form stated TURP. Of two patients who thought they may have had a prostatectomy, one had signed his consent form for a bladder neck incision and the other for a TURP and orchidectomy. One patient stated that he had had a prostatectomy but had signed for a TURP.

Operation described by women: D & C and hysteroscopy 5; did not know or did not remember 5; did not read the form 1; D & C, hysteroscopy and laparoscopy 1; D & C 4; D & C and clipped tubes 1; D & C, IUCD removal and sterilisation 1.

Comparing the women's consent forms with their statements we find that, of the seven women who gave the correct description, one who had signed for a D & C and hysteroscopy mentioned the D & C but not the hysteroscopy she had undergone; the consent form gave only D & C as the operation and the hysteroscopy was not mentioned. One patient, who identified D & C as the operation performed on her, had also undergone a hysteroscopy which was not mentioned on the consent form. Of those who were partially correct, one woman thought she had also had a laparoscopy, although she had not, and it was not mentioned on the form she had signed. Another woman knew of the D & C, the IUCD removal and the sterilisation but not of the hysteroscopy. Two who said only that they had had a D & C had also had a hysteroscopy, and one a polypectomy – both had signed consent forms for all these procedures. Another, who said she had had a D & C and clipped tubes, had in fact had the D & C and a laparoscopic sterilisation, but the consent form did not mention the D & C.

One woman thought the consent form was not filled in when she signed it, although she did in fact describe the same procedure as that mentioned on the form. Another woman stated that she should have had a laparoscopy but was told that as the operating theatre was not ready she did not actually have it; in fact there was no mention of laparoscopy on the consent form.

Clearly the comparisons show up a great deal of inconsistency and confusion.

4 Was there any other type of treatment available?

Answers: fourteen men said that no other kind of treatment was mentioned as being available, five said yes, and one said he did not know. Twelve women said no other kind of treatment was mentioned as being available, four said yes, one said that none was mentioned, and one was unsure.

Of the women who said that an alternative was mentioned two referred to 'the pill' and two to hysterectomy.

5 Were there any specific risks involved?

If the answer was yes, it was followed by the question: What were these risks?

Men's answers: there are no risks 13; none known to me 3; yes 1; yes, due to past or present medical condition 2; the usual operative risks 1.

Of the thirteen who stated there were no risks, one man replied, 'No, only sterility and sperm going into the bladder'; another that the only problem was needing repeat operations; and one said 'No. What risks?' The man who had suffered reactionary haemorrhage also said there were no risks.

Of the three patients who said they did not know of any risks, one stated that although he had not known of any before the operation his urinary catheter had become blocked by clots post-operatively so he now knew that was a risk. The one who answered yes said the risk was 'no sperm and smelly urine'. He had been told of these by a member of the medical staff pre-operatively. This same man had had a bacteraemic episode in the recovery room and although he knew that he had been shivering he did not know why.

Women's answers: no risks 7; yes, due to past or present medical condition 5; none read about 1; anaesthetic risk 1; assume there is a risk due to anaesthetic or haemorrhage 1; none or don't know 2; there could be 1.

Of the two men and five women who answered yes, due to past or present medical conditions, one had had bronchitis and the other a 'heart problem', but each told me he had not been told of the specific risks of TURP. One man and two women mentioned 'the usual' operative risks, i.e. risks associated with the anaesthetic and haemorrhage but said that they were not told of these by any of the staff.

6 Did you have ample opportunity to ask questions?

It was established whether the patient had in fact asked questions. Then I tried to establish whom they had asked.

Men's answers: yes 13; did not ask 1; not really 2; no 2; in too much pain to ask 2.

Of those who said yes, nine stated that the information came from doctors, one said it came from nurses and one said it came from doctors, nurses and ward charts. The patient who did not ask said, 'You trust the doctors.' One of those who said 'Not really' was the patient who had had the reactionary haemorrhage. He added, 'Doctors do not explain. Maybe they don't want you to know or are too busy. You just accept what you are told.'

Of the two men who said no, one did not think the junior staff knew enough about his surgery, and the other objected that 'one should not have to ask, all the information should be given'.

Women's answers: fourteen said yes; three said not really, and one said 'I think so'.

Of those who said yes, two had had a D & C before. Three of the patients said the information had come from doctors and nurses. One said she had been given a lot of information. Another said the information was sufficient but she did not have the courage to ask for more. Of three women who said 'not really', one was curious to know why her problems had gone on for so long but added that she was scared to ask and she thought the doctor would not have enough time anyway.

7 Do you remember signing a consent form?

If the answer was yes, it was followed by three further questions: a) Who asked you to sign the form? b) When did you sign the form? c) What is the consent form for?

Answers: nineteen men said they remembered signing the consent form and one that he did not; all the women said that they remembered.

a) Of the men, twelve said it was the doctor, five did not know, one was unsure and two that it might have been the anaesthetist. All eighteen women said it was the doctor who had asked.

b) Of the men, thirteen said they were asked the day before the operation, one on the day of the operation, four did not know, one said he could not now remember, and another said it was some time before the operation but was unsure when. Of the women, eleven said the day before the operation, five the day of the operation and two in the OPD.

c) Men: it gives permission to operate 4; not sure 3; no guarantee that operation will be performed by a specific person 2; to have the operation 4; to consent to be operated on to the extent necessary 2; to absolve them from trouble 1; don't know 1; to accept the operation, it's legally required for me to sign 1; consent for operation 2.

One man thought it might be to give consent to an injection. One of those who replied that it was permission to operate added that the doctors could not operate if the form was not signed. Another patient added that he could not 'come back on' the hospital if anything went wrong.

Women: to agree to have the operation 2; gives permission to do whatever they did do 3; it's a legal document 2; to agree to have the operation and that no specific person will carry it out 1; consent to have the operation 2; to give a free hand to investigate 1; to have a minor operation 1; allows them to do a hysterectomy or whatever if they find something else 1; if anything happens the doctor does not take responsibility 1; no idea 1; I must sign to have the operation 1; it tells you what the operation is and removes the hospital's responsibility 1; absolves the hospital from responsibility when they want to do anything else 1. The woman who said, 'I must sign to have the operation' could neither read nor write.

The replies to question 7c are grouped into types in Table 1.

Table 1 Replies to the question 'What is the consent form for?'

Kind of answer	Men	Women
Permission to operate	10	6
Carte blanche	2	4
Don't know	4	1
Absolves from responsibility	1	3
Legal requirement	1	2
No guarantee about surgeon	2	1
Allows free investigation	0	1

8 Did you read the consent form?

Men's answers: yes 4; no 7; a quick glance 2; I read some of the form 1; unsure 1; did not have reading glasses 2. (Three of the answers were not obtainable by this stage.) One of those who said no added, 'It's the law. There was no reason for me to read it.' One of those who did not have his reading glasses said the doctor had told him it was for the operation.

Women's answers: yes 11; no 6; didn't get the chance 1.

DISCUSSION OF RESULTS

The consent form

In the training of health care professionals much emphasis is put on the consent form as a document and on obtaining a signature on it for major treatments. In fact the form is only meant to provide some documentary evidence that an explanation of the treatment has been given and that informed consent has been sought and obtained. My research suggests that there was little or inadequately informed consent so that the signature in itself meant very little.

It is significant that 15 per cent of the patients interviewed did not even know what a consent form was for.

Men did less well than women in identifying the operation, thirteen of them stating that they did not know what operation was on the form even though I offered them three suggestions myself. Two of these (TURP and trans-urethral resection of the prostate) are in fact the same procedure, and the other is a prostatectomy which involves major abdominal surgery. Three thought they had had a prostatectomy and another two thought they probably had. (I regarded these as 'partially correct' in comparing the male patients' statements with consent forms, in question 3.)

One of the men I interviewed had signed for an operation of bladder neck incision which was different from the TURP he had actually had. Two of them had procedures other than a TURP, but these were not mentioned by the two men at interview.

It is possible that the women fared better because for them there was often a shorter delay between outpatient appointment and admission. Furthermore, the mean age of the men was 69.4 years and that of the women was 41.2 years. So it is likely that a difference in memory performance was also significant here. The age of the patient should be taken into account by nurses and doctors in the consent process. Much has already been written on the negative effects of age and anxiety on the memory, with recommendations on how to aid the older person to understand and retain the facts.[5]

However, the women also appeared to be somewhat vague or ignorant about the procedures that they signed for or underwent. One, woman who said only that she had had a D & C, had also signed for and had a hysteroscopy; another who said only that she had had a D & C, had also had a hysteroscopy which was not mentioned on the consent form; the woman who described her operation as a D & C and clipped tubes had actually had a laparoscopic sterilisation, as the consent form indicated, and a D & C which was not on the consent form.

In some cases it may be that patients are confused about what is part of a procedure and what is a separate procedure. Thus it is possible that some think that a hysteroscopy is a part of a D & C. This would be more likely to happen where an inadequate or no explanation had been given.

It is quite clear that in many cases incorrect or irrelevant information has been put on a consent form, or important information had been omitted. Thus three men had signed a consent form which included 'retrograde ejaculation' – which is not a treatment but one of the complications of a TURP.

It is disturbing that two of the male patients could not have read the consent form because they did not have their reading glasses with them, and neither said he had had the form read to him. Neither of them was an emergency admission. Nevertheless, one of the two was partially right in attempting to answer the question of what operation he had undergone.

The consent process

One may speculate that some of the discrepancies are to be explained by the forgetfulness or inattention of the patients. Some of these discrepancies can only be explained by shortcomings on the part of the staff. It may be that neither patients nor staff are taking consent as seriously as they should. A more comprehensive and rigorous study with a larger cohort, which I am preparing to undertake, should throw more light on the situation.

The process of consent which I described above requires a context of sufficient time and openness to allow the patient to ask questions and make a considered decision. A full explanation does not require that absolutely everything is conveyed to the patient but rather that the practitioner exercises skill and judgement in deciding what is important and relevant and how the information is conveyed. Furthermore, this is only one side of a relationship, for the patient too must be allowed to decide what is important and relevant. Thus there must be open and trusting conversation between patient and practitioner.

Questions 4, 5 and 6 were designed to examine the consent process in practice. The pattern which emerges supports the hypothesis that the patients were not well informed. Fourteen men and twelve women said there were no other treatments available. McLoughlin and Williams have recently reviewed the alternative treatments for growth of the prostate.[6] They conclude that at the present time alternatives to surgical intervention are limited and more research is needed in this area. It seems to me, however, that patients often like to know that there are no alternatives if there are none or that there may be an alternative treatment somewhere else or under development. Perhaps a questioning attitude on the part of patients would encourage more research into alternatives.

The picture for the women is slightly different, as the operation of D & C is performed as an investigative and diagnostic tool as well as a treatment. Even bearing this in mind it should still cause concern that only four of the eighteen women mentioned any alternative therapy such as the contraceptive pill or hysterectomy which had been discussed with them.

The patients' knowledge of the risks involved in the treatments was very limited, as we have seen. Actual risks involved in a TURP, as described by Winston and Mebust in 1988, include a mortality rate of 0.2 per cent, a failure to void of 6.5 per cent, bleeding in 3.9 per cent of cases, clot retention in 3.3 per cent, urinary infection in

2.35 per cent, urethral stricture in 2.5 per cent, and decreased sexual function at a rate closer to 4 per cent rather than 40 per cent.[7]

The risks involved in a D & C include post-operative infection, perforation of the uterus, and haemorrhage. Hysteroscopy risks include perforation of the uterus and bladder, infection, and fluid overload. Laparoscopy includes risks such as pain, puncture of abdominal organs and blood vessels, gas/air embolus and infection.

It is surely a matter for concern that not one of the patients interviewed mentioned any of the risks listed above. One man became aware of the risk of a blocked catheter only when it happened, and the man who bled so severely that he needed vaginal packs inserted was even then still oblivious of the risk of bleeding.

In addition to the surgical risks there are those associated with the patient being put in the lithotomy position. This requires the patient to lie on his back with his legs bent at the knees and hips and parted exposing the perineum area. This can cause pain and damage to the hip joints and thigh muscles, especially in patients with hip joint disease. This was in fact the case with the male interviewee who had post-operative pain.

Then there are anaesthetic risks, which were mentioned by two of the thirty-eight interviewees. These risks include drug and anaesthetic gas complications, equipment faults and human error. It is not customary for anaesthetists to explain these risks to patients, but some member of the surgical team should.

Reasons for not informing patients of specific risks, which may generally be offered by doctors, include: a) the doctor does not consider the risk to be important; b) the doctor appeals to 'benevolent concealment', that is, that in his/her judgement it would be in the best interest of the patient not to reveal some, or even any, of the risks. Both of these reasons might, if cogently justified, be upheld as decisive in a court of law.[8] A further reason which may be offered is: c) a lack of time and knowledge, which I think only really carries any weight in relation to junior doctors. I should have thought that the person obtaining consent always has a duty to make the time and to call someone more experienced if in doubt. It is interesting that three of the interviewees referred to this third possibility, although I should add that lack of time and knowledge does not absolve those responsible for obtaining consent.

The Department of Health guidelines state that those obtaining consent should take account of the possibility that the patient 'may be shocked, distressed or in pain'.[9] And we saw that four of the thirty-eight patients acknowledged that they were either in too much pain or too scared to ask for more information. The nursing staff carry out pre-operative checks to ensure that the correct patient arrives for the correct operation. More importantly they are, under the terms of their professional code, the advocates of their patients. Thus they have a special role in recognising anxieties and attempting to allay them as well as drawing the attention of the doctor to the fears and pain of the patient. In the study it emerged that either none of the nurses had noticed, or none of them took action after noticing, that three men had also consented to 'retrograde ejaculation', that one had signed the form for a bladder neck incision and had a TURP and that the man who had a reactionary haemorrhage seemed to know very little about what was happening to him.

The study suggests that the time at which consent is sought suits the convenience of staff rather than patients, and not enough time was allowed. If patients are to make a considered and informed decision they must be asked at the best time for them, and be given time to reflect, sort out their feelings and, if possible, discuss with spouses, friends or relatives. It is often said that there is insufficient time and a lack of trained personnel to follow such recommendations. But it should be kept in mind that the cost of not obtaining consent properly may cause suffering for the patient, complications and repeat operations and legal action.

The patient's notion of consent

The replies to question 7 indicate that patients see the signing of a consent form as a perfunctory and routine act to obtain their permission to proceed with treatment. Most did understand that their permission to operate was needed and that they had agreed that no guarantee could be provided about who would perform the operation.

Green reports that in a study 55 per cent of doctors and 79 per cent of patients thought that consent forms existed to protect doctors from a law suit, while 65 per cent of both groups thought the forms were to help doctor–patient communication.[10] Four of my interviewees thought that the consent form absolved 'them' (presumably doctors, hospitals, health authorities) from legal action. Some falsely thought a signed form gave the medical staff a 'free hand'. In fact the consent form cannot protect those responsible from legal action for negligence, and in any case it is *evidence* of informed consent which is legally significant, not the consent form in itself. A signed consent form is legally worthless where there is sound evidence that informed consent was not actually obtained.

None of my interviewees seems to have regarded the signing of the consent form as just one element in a joint decision making process. This suggests perhaps a passive attitude on the part of patients and a paternalistic attitude on the part of medical and other health care professionals. One suspects that the perceived 'authority' and 'expertise' of the professionals may evoke submissiveness on the part of patients which may in turn encourage high-handedness on the part of the professionals.

THE NURSING RESPONSIBILITY

It seems to me that this unsatisfactory situation arises in many British hospitals because the signing of the consent form is in practice an empty ritual, and little thought is given to consent as a process and a relation between patient and carer. The Department of Health guidelines state quite explicitly,

> It should be noted that the purpose of obtaining a signature on the consent form is not an end in itself. The most important element of a consent procedure is the duty to ensure that the patients understand the nature and purpose of the proposed treatment. Where a patient has not been given appropriate information then consent may not always have been obtained despite the signature on the form.[11]

The study suggests that the nursing staff did not understand their responsibilities, or did not act on them. It appears that the ward staff accepted the signatures on the operation consent forms even when the patients were unable to understand what the forms said, or the forms were wrong.

Some incidents I have witnessed are quite alarming. Both medical and nursing staff allowed a blind man's sister to sign the consent form for him, although the law does not recognise proxy consent except for a minor. What they did not seem to grasp was that it was the understanding of the treatment by the patient which was crucial. I did not include this patient in the study. In another case (included in this study), staff allowed an illiterate woman to put a cross on the consent form. Yet there is no health authority or hospital policy, or statement in the Department of Health guidelines, which supports such a practice. In fact, a witnessed oral consent would have been sufficient in both cases as long as the patient was properly informed and understood: 'Oral or written consent should be recorded in the patient's notes with relevant details of the health professional's explanation.'[12]

It is vital that nurses understand that the consent form is a permanent record of the treatment the patient has agreed to, and that it is as much their responsibility as the doctor's to ensure that informed consent is given.

The UKCC is very clear on this point in their 1984 advisory document 'Exercising Accountability'. First, the document points out that although in many instances it is the medical practitioner who seeks consent, the nurse should generally be present. 'Normally, in respect of patients in hospital, there are good reasons why the information should be given and the consent sought in the presence of a nurse, midwife or health visitor' (Sec. D 2). And, 'In certain situations and with certain client groups the [nursing] practitioner's level of responsibility in this respect is greatly increased where she stands in "loco parentis" for a patient or client' (Sec. D 3).

Here it is especially vulnerable groups, such as children, the elderly, the mental handicapped and the mentally ill which the UKCC has in mind. This point is, of course, connected with the professional duty, also emphasised by the UKCC, to act as the advocate of the patient.

Second, and more strongly, the attendant nurse has a duty to ensure that the consent procedure is followed. If there is a mishap or a patient complaint and the consent procedure was not followed then the attendant nurse is also responsible and may be liable:

> If the nurse, midwife or health visitor does not feel that sufficient information has been given in terms readily understandable to the patient so as to enable him to make a truly informed decision, it is for her to state this opinion and seek to have the situation remedied.
>
> (Sec. D 3)

So strong is the nurse's professional duty that she cannot absolve herself by simply proceeding on the ground that the doctor has insisted and she has to 'follow medical instructions'.

> The [nursing] practitioner might decide not to co-operate with a procedure if convinced that the decision to agree to it being

performed was not truly informed. Discussions of such matters between the health professionals concerned should not take place in the presence of patients.

(Sec. D 3)

The document goes on to recognise those situations, familiar to nurses, in which although the doctor has given an explanation the patient later turns to the nurse with a question, indicating that he or she did not really understand at all. 'Where this proves to be the case it is necessary for that [nursing] practitioner, in the patient's interest, to recall the relevant medical practitioner so that the deficiencies can be remedied without delay' (Sec. D 4). Although patients may not understand the biological details of some disease or dysfunction or a treatment this should not be used as an argument for not giving an adequate explanation particularly with regard to what consequences an intervention or non-intervention may have for a patient's life. Nurses are in a particularly good position to discuss consequences with the patient, which is vital if the patient is to decide on what course of action to follow.

CONCLUSION

Although I have emphasised consent as a procedure to be followed, I would not wish to encourage a defensive posture in nursing. It is more important to think of consent as a dialogue, and as a trusting relationship. Sherlock makes a case for a rethinking of consent as conceived in American law and medical practice. He says that it is not really procedural informed consent we should pursue but a relationship of mutual trust and respect.[13]

This non-defensive understanding of consent is much more in keeping with the goals and ideals of nursing.

NOTES

1 I am presently (1992–3) undertaking a larger and more detailed study of the same kind in several London hospitals.
2 Byrne, D. J., Napier, A. and Cuschieri, A., 'How Informed is Signed Consent?', *British Medical Journal*, 1988, vol. 296, pp. 839–40.
3 Department of Health, *A Guide to Consent for Examination and Treatment*, Heywood, Lancs.: Department of Health, 1990. On consent and the law also see Ann Young's chapter in this volume.
4 Dimond, B., *Legal Aspects of Nursing*, London: Prentice Hall, 1990, p. 254.

5 Morrow, G. R. *et al.*, 'Improving Physician–Patient Communications in Cancer Treatment', *Journal of Psychosocial Oncology*, 1983, vol. 1, pp. 93–101; Ley, P., 'Psychological Studies of Doctor–Patient Communication', in Rachman, S. (ed.) *Contributions to Medical Psychology*, vol. 1, Oxford: Pergamon, 1977, pp. 9–42; Simes, R. J. *et al.*, 'A Randomised Comparison of Procedures for Obtaining Informed Consent in Clinical Trials of Treatment for Cancer', *British Medical Journal*, 1986, vol. 293, pp. 1065–8; Sterling, E. D. and Yahne, C., 'Surgical Informed Consent: What it is and what it is not', *The American Journal of Surgery*, 1987, vol. 154, pp. 574–8.

6 McLoughlin, J. and Williams, G., 'Alternatives to Prostatectomy', *British Journal of Urology*, 1990, vol. 5, pp. 313–16.

7 Winston, K. M. and Mebust, M. D., 'Surgical Management of Benign Prostatic Obstruction', *Supplement to Urology*, 1988, vol. 32, pp. 574–7.

8 Dixon, E., *The Theatre Nurse and the Law*, London: Croom Helm, 1984; Kennett, A., 'Informed Consent: A Patient's Right', *The Professional Nurse*, December 1986, pp. 75–7; Wells, W. T., 'Medicine and the Law: The Surgeon's Duty to Warn of Risk', *The Lancet*, 28 April 1984, p. 974.

9 Department of Health, op. cit., p. 3.

10 Green, J. A., 'Minimizing Malpractice Risks by Role Clarification', *Annals of Internal Medicine*, 1 August 1988, p. 234.

11 Department of Health, op. cit., p. 4.

12 ibid.

13 Sherlock, R., 'Reasonable Men and Sick Human Beings', *The American Journal of Medicine*, 1986, vol. 80, pp. 2–4. See also Gutheil, T. G. *et al.*, 'Malpractice Prevention through the Sharing of Uncertainty: Informed Consent and the Therapeutic Alliance', *New England Journal of Medicine*, 1984, vol. 311, pp. 49–51; and Faulder, C., *Whose Body is it? The Troubling Issue of Informed Consent*, London: Virago Press, 1985.

Chapter 2

The observation of intimate aspects of care

Privacy and dignity

Paul Wainwright

INTRODUCTION

The impetus for this chapter comes from a discussion with a group of observers who were training to use an observation tool which required access to direct patient care. The tool in question was the Quality Patient Care Scale (Qualpacs), an instrument used to assess the quality of the process of care.[1] The tool involves observers watching the care given to a selected group of patients, identifying items of care from a checklist, and rating the quality of the performance of each item on a five point rating scale. The effective use of such a tool requires observers to position themselves so that they can 'both see and hear their selected patients. . . . It is permissible for assessors to enter behind screens to watch some aspects of care, provided that the patient has no objection.'[2]

Several trainee observers expressed discomfort at the intrusion into patients' privacy, required by the observation process. Objections raised centred on the duty to protect patients' privacy and dignity.

Research and quality assurance

There are many examples in the literature of quality assurance initiatives and research projects involving close observation of patient care, and reference to the question of privacy in many works on nursing research. Treece and Treece, for example, raise the issue, but come to no real conclusion other than to say that 'most guidelines for conducting research on human subjects are too vague' and noting that it is unclear what exactly is meant by 'invasion of privacy'.[3] They express the view that 'if privacy has been invaded, or moral or ethical issues are raised, the material should be published only after the subject has given his permission. A researcher should never betray the confidence of the subjects.'

Faulkner suggests that,

> pure observation, where the researcher chooses a position and simply notes what is happening around him/her, is unlikely to cause any ethical problems in most nursing situations. It can, after all, be argued that nothing underhand is going on. The observer only sees what everyone else sees.[4]

However, she goes on to challenge this assumption on the ground that some observation studies will require the observer to have knowledge of information such as the patients' diagnoses, which might require the consent of the patients concerned. Faulkner feels that observers are more likely to be criticised if the fact of their observation is concealed, as for example in participant observation.

The area of nursing research which provides the richest examples of the observation of care is that of nurse–patient interaction, and the following examples are among the better known. None is singled out here with the intention of suggesting that proper ethical procedures were not followed: they are offered to serve as a backcloth against which to reopen the debate about the moral issues involved.

Altschul's study of nurse–patient interaction in psychiatric units involved non-participant observation during which interactions between nurses and patients were timed and noted, and a full description of each interaction subsequently obtained from the nurse.[5] Stockwell investigated the extent to which nurses enjoyed caring for some patients more than others, and coined the phrase 'the unpopular patient' to describe those whom nurses found less attractive.[6] The study included non-participant observation of interpersonal behaviour and interactions between nurses and patients, and interviews with nurses to further explore their attitudes to nursing and to patients.

MacIlwaine asked female neurotic patients in psychiatric units of general hospitals to wear a radio microphone in order to record their interactions with nursing staff;[7] and Faulkner used a radio microphone to record nurse–patient conversations in a general hospital setting.[8] Macleod Clark describes using audio and video tape recordings to examine nurse–patient communication in surgical wards, and included in her data video film of pre-operative preparation and post-operative care, taking of temperature, pulse and respiration, drug rounds, dressings and admissions.[9] Bond studied nurses' communication with cancer patients, using direct observation of nurses in a way that allowed their conversations to be heard by the observer, and interviewing nurses after a conversation, so that they could report the content of the interaction to the researcher.[10] These studies, and others like them, raise many questions about the degree of access to intimate details of patient care which may be acceptable in the course of research.

The two quality assurance tools most often discussed in the UK literature are Qualpacs and Monitor.[11] Both require the direct observation of nurse–patient interaction by a non-participant observer. The use of Qualpacs has been mentioned above, and there are many more detailed accounts in the literature.[12]

Monitor requires some observation of care, although it also collects information from other sources, such as the nursing staff and the patients' records. In a discussion of difficulties experienced in the use of Monitor, Tomalin and colleagues note that to obtain answers to the questions in the instrument a continuous period of observation is often needed. They say, 'Some sources of information require considerable intrusion into a patient's privacy, particularly the questions that require observation of ostomies or catheters. This intrusion is exacerbated because the assessors, although nurses, are unfamiliar to the patients.'[13] In other instances the tool may require the assessor to question the patient about his or her experience of care.

While many writers recognise that observation has its difficulties its value is recognised. Dunne for example observes that, 'Many people involved in quality assurance feel that direct observation of nursing care is the most effective way of evaluating its quality and is critical to the success of the quality assurance programme.'[14] The objections raised by the Qualpacs trainees were presented in the context of individualised care, holistic approaches to nursing, and primary nursing. They reflect a contemporary shift in attitudes among many nurses towards their patients. This contrasts with those familiar anecdotes about practices in the past in which almost anybody might enter behind the closed screens around a patient, with barely a second thought.

The changing cultural situation brings to light a moral issue. Whatever the practices of the past it is increasingly recognised that patients should be allowed independence, including a right to privacy. In ordinary everyday social settings one expects to be afforded a certain level of privacy, when, for example, one is at one's personal toilet, but it is inevitable in the health care setting that there will be situations when patients will experience loss of privacy. In all but a few cases treatment as a patient will require an individual to expose him or herself to the scrutiny of others to an extent that would not be acceptable in normal social situations. Many patients will have to use communal toilet facilities and may have to sleep in rooms with other patients, while the process of assessment and diagnosis may require them to reveal their innermost thoughts and feelings, or to discuss intimate aspects of their lives with total strangers. However, the inevitability of such intrusions does not make them any more easily accepted or any less distressing to those involved; any reduction in privacy must be justified not just on grounds of practicality but also in terms of stronger moral claims.

At the same time there is a moral imperative to conduct research into clinical nursing practice, and to carry out exercises in quality assurance. These activities are necessary to ensure that patients have access to the best possible care and that knowledge about practice is increased or redirected. Research or quality assurance programmes may result in improvements in care for the patients involved, but more frequently any change in practice will only benefit future patients. Such activities are defended on the ground that the involvement of present patients will lead to the greater benefit of all patients.

Thus we appear to have two conflicting moral claims, and this gives us the dilemma: the obligation to respect human dignity by not intruding, and the obligation to advance nursing practice, which may necessitate intrusion.

It is not my intention to explore further the moral justifications for research and quality assurance: I will assume that in general they are necessary and have such justifications. However, there are occasions when one must question whether particular research or quality assurance activities are justified, in view of the intrusions into patients' privacy which they involve. This has been true for some time in the area of research, and in particular the research content of the curricula of many nursing courses. It is widely accepted that historically much of what passed for nursing knowledge was in fact derived from tradition, superstition, or trial and error, and when nurses were instructed in the techniques of their craft it was often considered more important that they accepted the authority of their instructors than that they should question the source of the knowledge.[15]

Quality assurance is a more recent phenomenon, having come to prominence with the introduction of general management in the 1980s. However, there is some evidence that the increase in quality assurance initiatives has not been without its problems, and one has to ask whether the consequent intrusion of privacy experienced by patients in areas subjected to various kinds of audit can be justified. If one is to defend such activities one must at the very least be confident that valid and reliable tools are being used by people who possess sufficient skills and knowledge. Examples of some of the problems associated with the imposition of quality assurance methods on staff and patients alike are discussed by Harvey and by Tomalin et al.[16]

The questions I wish to pursue are:

How are we to understand the concepts of 'privacy' and 'dignity'?
How does privacy relate to research, information and the professional role?
What are the moral objections to intrusion into intimate aspects of care by observers?
Are such objections so strong as to entail the prohibition of the use of such methods?

THE CONCEPT OF PRIVACY

One of the difficulties about any discussion of privacy is that, while most people can give some account of what they understand by the term, when we try to define it we find that its meaning is surprisingly unclear. As Scott says,

> While all of those who have written on the subject agree upon its fundamental importance to matters of human concern, that is about as far as the agreement has gone; it would be unquestionably difficult to formulate any more detailed thesis about the concept of privacy that would receive general approval.[17]

Scott points out that attempts to define privacy have dealt with it variously as a situation, a right, a claim, a form of control, or a value. It has been related to information, autonomy, identity, and physical access 'with a notable lack of coherence'.

The person

One area of agreement, according to Scott, is that all discussions of privacy link it with 'being a person' (human being, individual). Reiman, for example, says: 'privacy is a social ritual by means of which an individual's moral title to his existence is conferred'.[18] He goes on to suggest that privacy is an essential part of the process by which a social group recognises and communicates that an individual's existence is his own. To 'be a person' is to recognise not just one's capacity to shape one's destiny by making choices, but also one's exclusive moral right to shape one's destiny.

Parent defines privacy as 'the condition of not having undocumented personal knowledge about one possessed by others. A person's privacy is diminished exactly to the degree that others possess this kind of knowledge about him.' He goes on to discuss the nature of undocumented personal knowledge, suggesting that it consists in

> facts about a person which most individuals in a given society at a given time do not want widely known about themselves. They may not be concerned that a few close friends, relatives, or professional associates know these facts, but they would be very much concerned if the information passed beyond this limited circle.[19]

Facts of this sort might include a person's sexual preferences, drinking or drug habits, income, and the state of his or her marriage or health.

Information available from public records, such as newspapers and court reports, comes into the category of what Parent calls documented information. Thus to discover a man's criminal record from press reports is not to invade his privacy. On the other hand, information collected for special purposes and held in files such as medical records, is not in the public domain and steps are taken to ensure that there is no unauthorised access.

The body

Most accounts stress the importance of personal information and knowledge of, for example, one's innermost thoughts and feelings. Certainly, the revelation of one's thoughts and feelings to others, for example in the course of a medical consultation or nursing assessment, may threaten or diminish one's sense of one's self as an individual. None of these accounts make explicit reference to exposure of the human body as, in certain contexts, an invasion of privacy. However, in the context of the observation of intimate physical care this is important.

Revealing information about one's physical characteristics may be quite different from revealing the characteristics themselves. If a woman is in a labour ward about to give birth, her legs held apart in stirrups, and medical students unexpectedly enter, it is not as though she is troubled by their having gained personal information about her; she is troubled by what they have seen. In seeing her they may have probably gained no information at all, and yet from her point of view their seeing her in this way may be infinitely more offensive than all the information they might have gained about her.

Lawler points out that sensitivity about the private nature of the body and its functions is of great concern to nurses, who have to renegotiate socially the various norms, values, taboos, beliefs and learned ways of behaving with respect to the body.[20] She points out that the various disciplines that are concerned with the body and its functions use frameworks for their practice that are fundamentally mechanistic, reductive and empiricist, and which pretend to view the body 'objectively', as though it has nothing to do with personal matters. Lawler finds it necessary to marshal a variety of authorities to support the view that the body is integral to the person. Tacitly accepting a Cartesian dualism which she actually professes to reject, she argues that nurses are or should be concerned with integrating the 'object body' with the 'lived body' and stresses the importance of our understanding of the body as being closely interwoven with the person.

Lawler also quotes Elias' description of how since the eleventh century the body has been 'privatised' as society has shifted towards a more structured pattern of manners and more prescriptive patterns of beliefs, norms and values about the body, its functions and its products. According to Elias there has been a civilising process which has tended to make all bodily functions more intimate, and to put them behind closed doors, resulting in 'sociogenic shame and embarrassment'; many things associated with the body have become taboo.[21]

Weinberg's work shows how embarrassment about nudity depends very much on the rules embedded in a context. Thus nudists usually experience no embarrassment within the setting of the nudist camp, while the same nudism might be embarrassing in their own homes when visitors call. He suggested that it is possible to construct a system of rules to establish the context in which non-embarrassing nudism is possible.[22] Something similar is experienced more widely in the changing rooms of sports centres and swimming pools. Removing all one's clothes for the doctor or nurse may, of course, be somewhat embarrassing but it is strictly rule-bound and the way in which the parties act and what they say in such a situation is narrowly circumscribed for it to remain acceptable.

Professionals and inequality

Parent's account emphasises how privacy is determined by cultural norms and social practices. These practices include professional practices, of which nursing is one. There are also many situations in which we disclose personal information to selected individuals, such as bank managers, accountants, solicitors, clergymen, doctors, nurses, midwives, health visitors and social workers. The information is disclosed in the context of some kind of client relationship, which would usually give the individual some assurance of confidentiality. In most cases the information must be disclosed if clients are to receive a proper service from the professional concerned. This is not to say that all information divulged in the course of a professional consultation is freely given or is wholly necessary for a successful outcome: there is a considerable imbalance of power between professionals and their clients.

The extent to which such disclosure constitutes a loss of privacy is debatable. A person may feel that they have relinquished a restricted degree of their privacy in consulting a professional. However, it could be argued, in view of what Parent says about 'close associates', that disclosure under these conditions is not a loss of privacy at all. It would be regarded as curious to approach a professional for a service only to deny access to the information needed to provide the service, on the ground that it is private. Ordinarily a person goes to a professional with the attitude that certain information is not private as far as that professional is concerned, so there is no loss of privacy and certainly no invasion of privacy. Still, it is understandable if someone is reluctant to go to a professional in the first place because he or she has the attitude that such a relationship must involve a loss or invasion of privacy. Such reluctance may be more common in the field of human relationships, such as marriage guidance counselling or psychotherapy.

One should take into account the imbalance of power between patient and professional, be it the nurse or the doctor. Girard says 'One cannot help shuddering when one hears a "progressive" doctor insisting that she cannot treat a patient unless she knows everything about him' and he asks 'what authority, what validated science give her the right to force patients through a confessional?'[23] Girard points out that views of this nature are characterised as 'holistic', but claims that this model of the doctor–patient relationship tends towards a form of paternalism and that such paternalism is nothing less than a special form of medical sadism. Many critics of the 'nursing process' have objected to the introduction of comprehensive nursing assessments on similar grounds.

Girard argues that the dispenser and recipient of medical care experience a fundamentally unequal relationship. The patient may suffer incomprehension, be mentally, physically or psychically diminished, and experience or anticipate pain. The patient suffers what can be described as an 'ontological assault', is forced to place himself under the power of another person and is in a state of 'wounded humanity'. To suggest that a patient can continue to exercise his right of ownership and freedom of choice over disclosure, as he would if he were sharing information voluntarily with a close friend, may be naive. If the patient is coerced or compelled, by means of the imbalance of power in the relationship, to disclose information that is not required (according to Girard's 'scientifically validated' criterion) in order to contribute to diagnosis, treatment or cure, then it would seem that there has been a breach of privacy of the worst kind.

Clearly, anyone entering a hospital as a patient will be expected to disclose a considerable amount of personal information in the course of treatment. So long as certain restrictions (which I list below) are met, this disclosure will not generally be regarded as a loss of privacy. However, there is a very real possibility that a patient will suffer a loss of privacy by virtue of the conditions which still prevail in many hospitals. There are many reasons for this, not least the financial difficulties involved in upgrading old buildings built on the 'Panopticon' model (although, one should not forget, many patients still express a preference for multi-bedded rooms which provide company and companionship). However, unless patients have single rooms they will almost certainly have to reveal personal matters to other patients and their visitors.

Many hospitals have introduced a policy of mixed-sex wards, with patients accommodated in four- or six-bedded rooms, or with a larger ward area divided by partitions. In many of these wards patients of both sexes have to share bathroom and toilet facilities. As Elias has suggested, the civilising process at work in society over the last few centuries means that we do not normally disclose to others, except those closest to us, the state of our bowels or digestive system, or what we wear in bed, or that we have false teeth, or that we snore or break wind in our sleep. But when we share a hospital room or ward we have little option. We would usually prefer to consult our doctors and nurses without being overheard by strangers, and medical examinations can lead to some searching questions about our personal habits. We might prefer others not to see us *in extremis*, but even in death we may have little option but to reveal all to nearby strangers. Screens are not always available, and in any case are not soundproof.

OBSERVATION OF CARE

The nursing staff responsible for the care of a patient will have access to some personal knowledge about that patient and must have that access if they are to perform properly. From the professional point of view (and taking into account the reservations expressed above about the balance of power) this does not, if the restrictions are respected, necessarily involve any loss of privacy.

However, the involvement of non-participant observers is a different matter. An observer has no role in the care of particular patients and thus has no professional grounds for access. The presence of an observer must therefore result in a loss of privacy.

It could be argued that, just as patients have the right to consent to disclosure of information or knowledge to those directly involved in their care and that such controlled disclosure need involve no loss of privacy, so they have an equal right to decline to admit the observer. There are two practical problems. One is a continuation of the inequality argument already referred to. When the nurse who is responsible for the patient's care says, 'Do you mind if this other nurse comes to watch me work with you this morning – it is part of our quality assurance programme?', it takes a very strong patient indeed to refuse permission. The second is even more fundamental: does the patient actually recognise the distinction between the nurse who is caring for him or her, and the non-participant observer? Is the patient not more likely to assume that the observer is part of the hospital staff (as may be the case) and that he or she is therefore present by right, and that the request for consent to their presence is no more than a social nicety?

I have already argued that unless patients have rooms to themselves admission to hospital in most cases inevitably will result in a loss of privacy. Does the presence of an observer make any difference? I would argue that it does.

It might be held that, since privacy is a moral good, any act which results in the loss of it must be unethical, unless the right to privacy is overridden by some stronger moral demand. To take an extreme case, health carers have to assume that people would rather have their lives saved than their privacy respected, if a situation arose which presented that choice. Health carers certainly cannot assume the opposite, even if they later discover that the patient would in fact have preferred to be left privately to die.

Researchers engaged in observation may also be meeting a moral demand. They may intend that their research should lead to good ends, although in the case of non-therapeutic research these goods will not be brought to the subjects, but only to future patients, if ever. It is not at all clear whether the loss of privacy which results from research observations should be seen as a lesser consideration than the benefits which will or may accrue from the research. It is to be hoped that studies of the kind mentioned earlier have resulted in changes in the education of nurses, and thus in their practice, and that patients receive better care as a result. Similarly, quality assurance exercises may result in changes in management practice and even the allocation of additional resources to patient care areas, as a direct result of data gained through the observation process.

De-sensitisation and consent

In any event it seems wrong to argue that, just because the patient has already lost privacy, for example because of the presence of other patients, it would make no difference to allow access to an observer or observers as well. Nurses may not be able to achieve perfect privacy, but the point is that nurses have a duty to keep any loss of privacy to a minimum, by not allowing access to more people than they must.

The responsibility for safeguarding the privacy of patients must rest with all the staff involved, but I think a particular onus lies on the nursing staff of the ward or unit concerned. They have the ability to determine standards and develop management policies which minimise the number of people who have access to the patient, through such measures as skilful rostering and work assignment to provide continuity of care with a few nurses. Innovations such as primary nursing and the named nurse can help in this respect, but policies involving core staffing and the use of a multitude of part-time and bank or agency staff may have the opposite effect.

The nurse who is responsible for the patient also has a duty to look critically at questions such as visiting arrangements and the throng of students of the various health care professions who seek access to patients for educational purposes.

Privacy may be lost by degrees. There is a real danger that practical difficulties, sometimes rooted in under-resourcing and inappropriate administrative structures, lead to situations that nurses would prefer not to accept. After a time nurses become desensitised to a situation and it becomes the norm. Circumstances then occur which lead to a further (temporary) deterioration in standards, and the nurses and other professionals become accustomed to the new norm. Some of the scandals of the past, involving long-stay hospitals for the elderly or mentally ill, no doubt resulted in part from this kind of habituation.

The usual way to try to overcome the kind of difficulties I have described is to seek the patient's consent to the presence of an observer. Such a request would normally be accompanied by some explanation of the reason for making the observations, together with assurances of anonymity or confidentiality. Is this sufficient?

The patient who agrees to allow access to an observer will be giving consent to some loss of privacy, in whatever degree may be demanded by the nature of the study. Of course, to speak of 'degrees of privacy' implies that privacy and its loss can be measured on some kind of ordinal scale, but it must be virtually impossible for the subject who is to be observed to anticipate in any precise way just how embarrassed he or she may be in the situation to which they are asked to consent. One cannot truly consent to what one cannot anticipate. However, the observers should no doubt always make some effort to put themselves in the shoes of the subjects so as to go some way to being in a position to explain to them what might be involved.

In any case, it is because of such dangers of embarrassment and affront to patients, and the difficulties in knowing precisely what will cause these reactions, that researchers and those who engage in quality assurance exercises must be able to state with cogency that the proposed project is justifiable in terms of its benefits.

Dignity

That a patient will, or may, be made to feel undignified by some behaviour or course of action on the part of nurses and other health carers is sometimes sufficient to throw that behaviour or course of action into question. A dictionary will define 'dignity' in terms such as these: 'Nobility of aspect, manner or style; becoming stateliness, gravity.'[24] Dignity is perhaps too strong a word, 'self-esteem' being more appropriate in most contexts.

It is false dignity, or a sudden shedding of dignity, which are so often the main element in comedy, such as pantomime, farce and slapstick. Jokes about people who are odd in aspect, manner or style, about falls, or certain bodily functions and clothing, achieve their humorous effect partly because they are undignified. If we look for equivalent situations in hospital we may think of procedures such as enemas, injections, bed baths and sigmoidoscopies – all of which have featured in crude jokes, cartoons and films. Men undergoing vasectomy have described the indignity of being draped for the operation.

One reason that patients are made anxious by such situations is that they may feel that they are being exposed to ridicule. This is as true of the man who has to lie with his shaved genitals poking through a hole in a green cloth as of the one who slips on a banana skin on the pavement. But ridicule requires a further element: the presence of observers bearing a certain attitude. If I slip on the ice and no one is watching I may not feel ridiculous; and if someone is watching but offers only genuine concern I may not.

Many aspects of intimate care come into the category of undignified or potentially undignified situations, which may threaten to become ridiculous ones. The kind of care or treatment which involves the nurse working behind closed screens, or in the bathroom, toilet or treatment room, frequently requires the exposure of parts of the body not usually revealed to strangers, or which require the patient to adopt an ungainly or unseemly posture, or to reveal the extent of his or her dependence on help with basic activities.

One way to overcome or minimise a loss of dignity or self-esteem is for those involved to treat the situation with dignity themselves, maintaining an appropriate distance. There has been an increasing tendency of late to criticise a concentration on the technical aspects of care as evidence of a reductionist and, it is implied, an uncaring approach to the patient. However Girard suggests that 'the patient's necessary abandon [has] somehow to be limited' and calls for a 'more complex form of reserve: an emotional and intellectual chastity'. For Girard the fundamental question of medical ethics is 'how to establish with precision the distance to which a patient is entitled in order to feel respected and recognised'. Girard recognises that the technical model has the potential danger of a dehumanisation of medicine. However, he argues that the extent of our scientific knowledge or technical power provides us with an upper bound of what can be done with a patient and he concludes that the concept of technical expertise as an ethical form needs to be reappraised.

Thus, the presence of individuals who, far from showing ridicule, contempt or distaste, treat the matter as one that is serious and that requires their professional and technical skill and attention, can help to maintain the patient's dignity and overcome any sense of an invasion of privacy. Just as the health care workers involved in performing a task can retain a sense of dignity or decorum, so an observer can do the same. This can be achieved by maintaining a neutral expression and demeanour, being careful about body language, avoiding eye contact and generally adopting a serious manner focused strictly on the health care matters at hand.

Special groups

I have discussed the issues of privacy and dignity in very general terms. There are, however, some groups of patients who present special problems, although I do not have space to examine them in detail here.

Children are frequently disregarded, or assumed not to have any legitimate views on their involvement in research or other projects, but are, I would submit, just as entitled to privacy and dignity, and just as much at risk of harm from disregard of these rights, as adults are. Children are quite capable of expressing an opinion or a preference from a very early age, and the legal age of consent should not be taken to mean that children below the age of 16 years need not be consulted.

Pregnant women, and particularly those in labour, are another vulnerable group, with ever-increasing numbers of students and trainees from occupations only remotely connected with health care seeming to think it essential that they observe antenatal sessions and deliveries.

The elderly, especially those with dementia and other mental health problems associated with ageing, seem to have their privacy disregarded by all and sundry, to a regrettable extent. We still hear stories of patients or residents of homes being expected to use commodes in public places, or left until they have been incontinent where they are sitting and then cleaned up in a public way.

The mentally ill and mentally handicapped are subjected to public scrutiny in a variety of ways which amount to a severe loss of privacy and dignity or self-esteem. Indeed, it could be argued that the patients discharged from mental institutions into the community, without adequate provision of accommodation and protection, lose whatever vestige of privacy and dignity their seclusion in an asylum may have afforded them.

CONCLUSION

The presence of a non-participant observer does threaten a loss of privacy or dignity for the patient concerned. It may also result in such a loss for any other patients who may not themselves be involved in the study but who can be seen or heard by the observer. However, this can be either completely or largely overcome.

1 Health carers and observers should seek the free and informed consent of the patients involved and others who may be affected. In particular, the patients should understand the purpose of the observation and be assured that they are free to ask for the withdrawal of the observers without any detrimental effect on their subsequent care.

2 Loss of dignity can be avoided if those involved maintain a serious and respectful manner towards the patients and carers involved.

3 It is essential that proposals for observation exercises go before ethical review committees, and that these committees always keep in mind the possible loss of privacy for, and affront to the dignity of, the patients concerned.

I also suggest here some conditions under which the disclosure of personal information, in the context of a client–professional relationship, might take place:

1 *Restricted scope*: The information collected should be that which is required to enable professionals to carry out their functions. To gather personal information about the client which bore no relationship to the matter at hand would be an invasion of privacy.

2 *Restricted access*: Reasonable steps should be taken to restrict access to the information collected to those who need it by virtue of their involvement in the case. This is likely to include professional colleagues, but may also include secretarial and support staff.

3 *Restricted use*: Personal information collected for the purpose of providing a professional service to the client should not be used for other purposes not authorised by the client.

In my view these conditions provide the minimum safeguards required to protect the privacy of an individual. Any deviation from or extension beyond these restrictions would require justification on moral grounds that outweigh the basic requirement of respect for privacy. Such restrictions do not preclude the use of observation techniques, for research or quality assurance, but they do require that such exercises are subjected to proper ethical scrutiny and that adequate grounds can be given for the collection of the information involved.

NOTES

1 Wandelt, M. and Ager, J., *Quality Patient Care Scale*, New York: Appleton Century Crofts, 1974.

2 Wiles, A., 'Quality of Patient Care Scale', in A. Pearson (ed.), *Nursing Quality Measurement*, Chichester: John Wiley & Sons, p. 29.

3 Treece, E. W. and Treece, J. W., *Elements of Research in Nursing*, St Louis: The C. V. Mosby Company, 1977, pp. 39–40.

4 Faulkner, A., 'Nursing as a Research Based Profession', *Nursing Focus*, August 1980, p. 477.

5 Altschul, A., *Patient–Nurse Interaction: A Study of Interaction Patterns in Acute Psychiatric Wards*, Edinburgh: Churchill Livingstone, 1972.

6 Stockwell, F., *The Unpopular Patient*, London: Royal College of Nursing, 1972.

7 MacIlwaine, H., 'The Communication Patterns of Female Neurotic Patients with Nursing Staff in Psychiatric Units of General Hospitals', in J. Wilson-Barnett (ed.), *Nursing Research: Ten Studies in Patient Care*, Chichester: John Wiley & Sons, 1983, pp. 1–24.

8 Faulkner, A., 'Monitoring Nurse–Patient Conversation in a Ward', *Nursing Times*, 30 August 1979, pp. 95–6.
9 Macleod Clark, J., 'Nurse–Patient Communication: an Analysis of Conversations from Surgical Wards', in J. Wilson-Barnett (ed.), op. cit., 1983, pp. 25–56.
10 Bond, S., 'Nurses' Communications with Cancer Patients', in J. Wilson-Barnett (ed.), op. cit., 1983, pp. 57–79.
11 Harvey, G., 'An Evaluation of Approaches to Assessing the Quality of Nursing Care Using (Predetermined) Quality Assurance Tools', *Journal of Advanced Nursing*, 1991, vol. 16, pp. 277–86.
12 Wainwright, P. J., 'Qualpacs – a Practical Guide', in *The Ward Sister's Survival Guide*, London: Austen Cornish Publishers Ltd, 1990, pp. 171–5.
13 Tomalin, D. A., Redfern, S. J. and Norman, I. J., 'Monitor and Senior Monitor: Problems of Administration and Some Proposed Solutions', *Journal of Advanced Nursing*, 1992, vol. 17, p. 76.
14 Dunne, L. M., 'Quality Assurance: Methods of Measurement', *The Professional Nurse*, March 1987, p. 188.
15 Since the Briggs Report there has been concern that nursing should become a 'research based profession', with the result that almost every course contains some discussion of research method, and there have been many courses created in what has become known as research awareness or appreciation. Unfortunately, teachers seem to be of the view that in order to gain an understanding of the importance of research, it is essential that students have themselves some experience of the practicalities of data collection, and this has led to a considerable increase in the number of so-called research projects being conducted by students, often in ways that are wholly inappropriate and without adequate instruction or supervision. See Department of Health, *Report of the Committee on Nursing*, London: DHSS, 1972, p. 108.
16 Harvey, op. cit.; Tomalin et al., op. cit.
17 Scott, G. E., *Moral Personhood*, Albany: State University of New York Press, 1990, p. 132.
18 Reiman quoted in Scott, op. cit., p. 134.
19 Parent, W. A., 'Privacy, Morality, and the Law', in J. C. Callahan (ed.), *Ethical Issues in Professional Life*, New York: Oxford University Press, 1988, p. 216.
20 Lawler, J., *Behind the Screens: Nursing, Somology, and the Problem of the Body*, Melbourne: Churchill Livingstone, 1991, p. 1.
21 Elias quoted in Lawler, op. cit., pp. 73–4.
22 Weinberg quoted in Lawler, op. cit., pp. 138–9.
23 Girard, M., 'Technical Expertise as an Ethical Form: Towards an Ethics of Distance', *Journal of Medical Ethics*, 1988, vol. 14, pp. 25–30.
24 *Shorter Oxford English Dictionary*, Oxford: Oxford University Press, 1980.

Chapter 3

Choice and risk in the care of elderly people

Linda Smith

Although many elderly people need care to a greater or lesser bn degree it is erroneous to believe that all elderly people will become dependent.[1] Unfortunately, there is a tendency in British society to regard old age as a totally negative experience and to perceive elderly people as burdensome and unproductive. Townsend puts forward the view that modern British society structures the dependency of older people and creates a climate in which elderly people are forced into a disadvantaged position which creates a need for support.[2]

Nurses who, in their working lives, meet only elderly people who are sick, frail or cognitively impaired have a strongly reinforced image of the hopelessness and helplessness of old age. These attitudes often lead the nurse to adopt a paternalistic stance towards her/his patients with a subsequent erosion of the patients' independence.

Nurses, together with other professionals, frequently make decisions without consulting with the elderly patient. Even when patients do make their wishes known they are largely ignored, the professionals believing that they know what is best. In many cases the quality of life for elderly patients is reduced to an untenable degree.

I shall look at a number of case studies to explore the issue of elderly patients' independence, and their freedom to take risks and even choose death. I shall relate this issue to the 'competence' of patients and the paternalistic conformism of nurses.

INDEPENDENCE

In 'Western' society it is now generally held that we should respect others as individuals who have a right to determine their own lives so long as they do not interfere with the rights of others. Nurses often see themselves as being in the difficult position of deciding whether an older person in their care is capable of making reasonable decisions about their lives, and also whether the older person's wishes and actions will place an unbearable load upon those who will be responsible for providing care.

The UKCC Code of Professional Conduct states in its first two clauses that each nurse, midwife or health visitor shall:

1 Act always in such a manner as to promote and safeguard the interests and well-being of patients and clients.
2 Ensure that no action or omission on your part, or within your sphere of responsibility, is detrimental to the interests, condition or safety of patients and clients.[3]

Clearly, the nurse should do what is good for the patients and avoid anything that will harm them. One of the reasons that elderly people are deprived of choice is that nurses are frequently caught by the dilemma that it would be good, for example, to help the elderly to return home (which is usually their overriding desire), but to do so might cause them to come to harm due to their age-related impairments.

The case of Elsie

Elsie was 91 years old when she was admitted with a severe chest infection to a unit for care of elderly people.[4] When found by a neighbour her house had been cold and untidy, and Elsie was ill in bed. *In extremis* she had soiled the bedclothes and floor. She had been living alone for many years, since the death of her husband, and having no living relatives her social interactions had been mainly confined to her immediate neighbours and the local shopkeepers.

The multidisciplinary team in the hospital had formed the opinion that her ability to care for herself was severely compromised and it was suggested that she consider moving into a residential home. This suggestion was adamantly rejected by Elsie. The nursing staff continued to extol the virtues of the trouble-free living which would be provided by residential care. In fact, the social worker had already begun the process of finding a suitable home for Elsie to be offered when she was 'in a better frame of mind'.

One day Elsie asked that I (her nurse) read to her because her sight was so poor and, feeling that this might be an opportunity to broach the subject of her future yet again, I sat down to read a magazine. One of the stories in it was that of a family who had sold up all their property and bought a yacht in preparation for a round-the-world trip. When I had finished reading I remarked that some people took terrible chances, to which Elsie replied laughing that she was in more danger making a cup of tea. She added that life was always 'a gamble which sometimes you win and sometimes you lose'. Elsie then kept me spellbound with stories of her youth, the war, her husband's love of fast cars, the time they were lost on Ben Nevis in a snowstorm and how, just before her husband's death eighteen years ago, they had used all their savings to visit Japan, which had always been a dream of theirs.

As I listened I realised that Elsie, far from being unaware of our machinations, was trying to make the point that to end such a life in a home was totally alien to her nature.

She finished by touching my hand kindly and saying that she knew we meant well but that if she went into a home she would probably die of boredom, and that even if she did fall or get ill at home it was better than a passive existence in a strange place. Elsie eventually did go back to her own home with the provision of social services. I do not know how she managed, but I do know that in this case it was right that she was helped to take the chance.

Reflections on Elsie

When considering Elsie's story, a story which most nurses who care for elderly people will find familiar, several points arise. Her character, intelligence and experience made it possible for her to stand her ground against pressure which another elderly person may have found unbearable. The elderly people of the present matured at a time when doctors and nurses were rarely questioned. The practice of medicine was surrounded by a mystique which professionals did little to dispel. The word of the doctor or nurse was regarded as Gospel truth and to question it would have been considered disrespectful. In addition, elderly people in many cases would have absorbed a view of society in which their opinions held

little value, believing that they should gratefully accept whatever
was offered.

Research has found that nurses frequently exhibit paternalistic
behaviour,[5] and even when patients try to speak of anxieties they are
often ignored (perhaps because many nurses really feel impotent in
the face of the patient's problems). The 'nurse knows best' is a view
held by nurses themselves. What chance then is there for an elderly
person to make decisions?

Consider this in contrast with a typical unit which cares for young
accident victims who have suffered paraplegia or quadriplegia. In
such a unit, from the moment of admission the objective of the
professionals is to help that person to return to whatever independence is possible. It could be argued that a young man who is
paralysed from the neck down, confined to a chair and in need of
assistance to breathe is taking far more risks out in the community
than someone like Elsie, but his right to take them is rarely
questioned. Is this because he is young?

What Elsie's case shows is that each of us has a vision of what his
or her life is or should be, of what makes it worthwhile. How people
should lead their lives cannot be determined on medical or nursing
criteria. For many people a dependent life is not a life really worth
living.

TAKING RISKS: FALLS

Falling accidents are extremely common on wards for the care of
elderly people. Certainly, British nurses are now becoming more
aware of the legal implications of accidents in hospital. Grant and
Hamilton say, 'physicians, nurses, health related personnel and
health care institutions are at risk of incurring financial losses if
these patients or their family members resort to court action to
recover compensation from the fall'.[6] There is a danger here that to
protect themselves against litigation health care professionals will
further curtail the freedom of movement of patients.

In Askham's comprehensive review of the research into falling
accidents, it is clear that studies have shown that elderly people are
more likely to fall when in institutions.[7] Most hospitals have an
accident reporting system which, though primarily designed to
ensure that appropriate care is given, often appears threatening or
'blaming' to the nurse involved. This might be the reason that nurses
often feel unable to let patients take any risks at all. Redfern says

that, 'The fear of accident so often takes precedence that nurses, other health workers, and relatives at home overprotect the old person and inadvertently assist the vicious cycles.'[8] An example of the vicious cycles she refers to is that involved in confining patients to beds and chairs and so on for 'their own good'. But this compromises their rehabilitation, which is not for their own good.

The case of John

John was a 79-year-old retired army sergeant who had suffered a right cerebro-vascular accident. He had some movement in both his left arm and leg but the movements were uncontrolled. He proved to be a strong and determined man who was fond of saying that neither the war nor the army had beaten him so this stroke would not.

As John's rehabilitation progressed the anxiety of the nurses increased. He refused to wait for assistance. The stack of accident forms grew and after numerous falls he took on the appearance of a prize fighter with a black eye, a sutured forehead and numerous other bruises.

No amount of pleading, discussion, scolding or inducement made the slightest difference. John's wife tried to make him 'see reason' but gave up eventually, telling the nurses he had always been 'headstrong'. The nurses considered cot-sides, a confining chair, removal of his walking frame and even a request for tranquillising drugs to be prescribed. Fortunately, with some courage, the staff decided against all these measures and instead ensured that John's shoes were appropriate, that he was placed in a position near the bathroom and that a close watch was kept on him to avert as many falls as possible.

John took only eight weeks to regain enough mobility to walk out of the ward, his wife proudly by his side.

Reflections on John

John was lucky to be on a ward where the nurses had already adopted a 'holistic approach' and were confident enough to give him his freedom to take risks in spite of the very real possibility that he could do himself serious harm. Obviously, they were reluctant to do this at first, and although this reluctance is questionable it is quite understandable under the present legal and administrative circumstances of care.

In the end what was important was John's character and outlook on life. It was accepted that to confine him may have risked breaking his spirit entirely and the outcome could have been very different. Like Elsie he was assertive and able to make his views known. There are many patients who would have succumbed to pressure: 'stay still', 'wait for us to come', 'don't try to walk on your own' and so on. Many nurses would have employed chemical or physical restraint to solve the 'problem'. What is needed is an environment of care and a nursing attitude which goes beyond allowing 'exceptions' like Elsie and John to the wider presupposition that all patients want greater freedom, so that it is the ones who do not or cannot who are the exceptions.

CHOOSING DEATH

If we accept that in general nurses should practise on the assumption that patients should determine their own lives in accordance with their own values, even or especially when sick or disabled or elderly, then not only should less emphasis be put on risk but patients' wishes regarding their own death should be respected too. This is not to say there are no exceptions or special circumstances, of course.

All nurses who work with elderly people will have experienced patients who express a wish to die and refuse treatment which may prolong their lives. Even if it is granted in principle that patients have a right to refuse treatment, or food, this will often depend on some judgement about the patient's 'competence' and this is made by the doctor. Kennedy maintains that in actual practice,

the law is constructed in such a way that very probably only the lucid and self-assertive patient who has a sympathetic and understanding doctor is able in most circumstances to have his own way and to be left alone in freedom to die. All other patients run the risk of having their wishes flouted.[9]

I shall now look at three cases, which are rather different from one another: Agatha, Doris and Arthur.

The case of Agatha

Agatha was a woman of 77 years who had severe rheumatoid arthritis, was in continuous pain and who, because of a severe deformity, was confined to a bed on a continuing care ward. She was washed, fed and turned regularly.

She enjoyed watching television and listening to music and had a good relationship with the nurses. She endured her life for three years until one day she said that she would like to be helped to die.

Her heart and lungs were strong, no pressure sores had developed, she had no urinary tract infections and was able to eat and drink.

Agatha lived for two more years before her death due to stroke. Throughout that period she would, at least once a week, ask for help to die.

The case of Doris

Doris was 98 years old, incontinent and hemiplegic with a small pressure sore on her hip. She had previously had a quite good appetite but over a period of time she began to refuse most of her food. For a time she would willingly take only tea or fruit juice, but eventually she refused even these. She became thin and dehydrated.[10]

A nasogastric tube was inserted, and Doris promptly pulled it out. Further attempts were made and each time she pulled it out. The nurses decided to make a pair of mittens from bandages and wool and these prevented any further removal of the tube.

Doris eventually died in spite of tube feeding. There was no obvious cause of death, although chest infection was recorded as the cause.

Reflections on Agatha and Doris

Agatha's condition was distressing to her and her carers. While the moral difficulties created by her case are perhaps even more acute than Doris' case, the legal situation is clearer. Complying with the choice she had made would have raised the problems of active euthanasia. She did not attempt to starve herself to death, but was suggesting that those caring for her take action to end her life. To ask carers to do this, though quite understandable in view of her condition, was to ask them to break the law and commit murder.[11]

The legal constraints do not, of course, resolve the moral issue. Some would argue that the law is wrong.

Whereas we clearly know what Agatha wished for, but would be unable to act on it without breaking the law (assuming such action is morally acceptable, which is controversial) in Doris's case we cannot even be sure what she wants. Was Doris's gradual refusal to eat an indication that she wished to die or was it a symptom of her deteriorating physical condition? More simply, it may have been her response to an irritating object in her nose and throat. (Nasogastric tubes are generally very uncomfortable.)

Should the nurses and doctors have considered whether there was any real point in striving to keep Doris alive? Here we are not talking about active euthanasia, but of allowing her to die. She was 98 years old, had suffered a severe stroke, and was deteriorating rapidly. The decision could have been made, in consultation with the relatives, to let dying take its course unhindered, ensuring at all times of course that Doris suffered no pain or unnecessary discomfort – that her mouth was clean and her skin intact and that offers of food and drink were made regularly. The nasogastric tube and, worse, the mittens, almost certainly increased her discomfort and made her last days of life very unpleasant. The mittens were seen as being necessary to circumvent a certain 'risk'. (In fact, the fitting of mittens brings new risks because excessive sweating combined with pressure can initiate the formation of sores and contractures.)

When nurses try to think about what their role is, surely they must consider that, besides responsibilities for helping patients to return to a state of health and for rehabilitation and adaptation to altered physical states, they also have responsibilities in helping dying patients make choices, even 'risky' ones, to achieve as peaceful, pain-free and dignified an end as possible. In the case of those with diagnosed terminal diseases acceptance of this role is not so difficult perhaps. But nurses should also consider their responsibility to achieve the same ends for people like Doris, whose condition is less well defined.

The case of Arthur

Arthur was 80 years old and was admitted with Parkinson's disease, a urinary tract infection, a chest infection and cataracts. He stated from the day of his admission that he felt his life was unbearable. Even when not suffering infections his blindness and the enforced

immobility of his Parkinson's disease limited his life to such an
extent that he no longer wished to continue it.

The nurses caring for Arthur listened to him. Good relationships
had developed with his loving family and they also felt that his
choice should be respected. The medical staff, when approached
with this idea, refused even to consider stopping treatment.

Arthur's condition worsened and he frequently wept as he repeated his wish. The doctors inserted an intravenous cannula to
maintain hydration. Arthur then submitted to a nasogastric tube,
saying that it was pointless to argue. Intravenous antibiotics were
given.

The senior nurse and her qualified staff continued to make their
opinion known that non-intervention would be the right thing, but
treatment was continued.

After three weeks, to everyone's surprise, Arthur's condition
began to improve. His infections responded to the medicines and
the symptoms of Parkinson's disease were alleviated by a new drug
regime. Arthur began to adopt a more positive demeanour and after
a further four weeks he was able to go home. He visited the ward a
year later having had the cataracts successfully removed. He
thanked everyone for saving his life.

Reflections on Arthur

The nurses who cared for Arthur were, of course, pleased by the
happy outcome of his treatment, but the episode caused much heart
searching among them. Some were quite worried that they had
made 'a mistake' and that the medical staff had been proved right.
The sister of the ward even expressed the view that she felt that she
would never again feel confident enough to make such a stand on
behalf of a patient, for fear of 'condemning to death' a person who
might have had the opportunity of satisfactory living for several
more years.

The medical staff (not without some smugness) felt that they had
been justified in ignoring the opinions of the nursing staff. In fact
this view of theirs extended to other areas of nursing care such as
wound management and preparation for discharge. As far as I
know, the medical and nursing staff never got round to discussing
the unilateral decision to continue the treatment. This case says a lot
about medical and nursing attitudes. The doctors should have
considered the options in discussion with patient, relatives and

nurses and given reasoned arguments for the proposed treatment. Arthur, and his relatives, could have had explained to them the possibility of a good outcome of treatment. They could have been asked to give the professionals a set period of time (say a month) to do what they could, and if at the end of the period Arthur was no better then consideration could be given to cessation of treatment. In this way Arthur might have felt more positive about his condition knowing that one way or another it would be addressed. Giving information, consulting and 'negotiating' in this way are quite commonplace in oncology units, but are still relatively rare in wards for elderly people. Nurses need to grapple with such situations and accept that being accountable does not mean that mistakes can never be made.

'COMPETENCE'

No doubt the paraplegic young man, whom I mentioned earlier, fully understood his situation or, in medico-legal language, was 'mentally competent'. But one of the difficulties of caring for elderly people is that there is more likelihood of cognitive failure occurring. Conditions such as Alzheimer's disease, long-term hypoxia due to chest or heart disease, and arteriosclerosis causing confusional states and depressive illness are not uncommon in the elderly. Such patients may have difficulty in understanding what is going on around them. It has been said that when considering decision making the professional sometimes has to decide whether the patients are 'competent' to make decisions. Many writers in medical ethics have, with difficulty, tried to formulate a list of criteria for establishing 'competence'. These sometimes derive from legal standards, and Beauchamp and Childress have suggested combining these standards thus:

> A person is competent if and only if that person can make reasonable decisions based on rational reasons. In biomedical contexts this standard suggests that a competent person is able to understand a therapy or research procedure, to deliberate regarding major risks and benefits, and to make a decision in light of this deliberation.[12]

I think nurses, as the advocates of patients, have to be careful with this concept of 'competence'. So often it serves paternalistic ends and medical power. 'Competence' suggests some technical or scientific way of establishing what freedom to allow another person. It is better perhaps to speak of 'understanding', which is a matter of judgement based on a personal, rather than merely professional, relationship.[13] Unfortunately, all too often nurses who care for elderly people take decision making out of the hands of patients who do meet these criteria simply because they have become used to doing so for those who do not meet them. Also, nurses sometimes assume that because a patient is unable to carry out one task, or a certain range of tasks, they are unable to carry out the one relevant to the decision at hand.

In the light of the above, let us consider the plight of those patients who, due to catastrophic physical degeneration, have to live out their lives in continuing care wards. Although there is a high percentage of such patients who suffer from dementia, there are many who are only physically disabled. In these cases often the few decisions they are able to make are not considered. What to wear, what to eat, how to spend leisure time, when to get up or go to bed or whether to have a bath or not are decided by the staff, usually to fit in with ritualistic routines which do not reflect a modern approach to nursing. It is all too easy to justify such routines on the ground that patients are not 'competent'.

The case of Emily

Emily was a patient who had been admitted to a continuing care unit after suffering a right brain stroke which had been followed some weeks later by a left brain stroke. She was confined to a chair, incontinent, and aphasic. Emily's only utterance was 'gid', which she used in response to all attempts at communication. It seemed that Emily could inject a wealth of meaning into this word of hers. It could be used angrily, 'GID! GID!'; as a question, 'Gid?'; as an urgent request for attention, 'Gid-gid-gid-gid!'; with a smile as a greeting, or with a tear of sadness.

Despite this demonstration of some understanding, of being able to put things in emotional context, Emily was usually treated by the nurses as being demented and her attempts at communication were often viewed with amused tolerance.

Due to her strokes Emily was only given soft foods, for fear that she would choke. The nurses on her previous ward had identified a severe dysphagia and, without attempting to assess her further, the unit staff had continued to feed her mince and fish. Emily was prone to dramatic temper tantrums, which usually occurred when she was being bathed, at meal times and at bed times. The nurses' way of handling this was to ignore the behaviour entirely and continue with whatever they were doing.

Emily was usually spoon-fed in her armchair away from the dining table because she would often shout or spit or push the food onto the floor. One particular day a new agency nurse, who was not used to the routine, pushed Emily's chair to the table next to a patient who ate a normal diet. The food on the menu that day was chicken drumsticks. Emily had partial use of her right hand and arm and with the speed of light she snatched her neighbour's drumstick and took a large bite. The permanent staff, on seeing what had happened, rushed to deal with what they felt would be an inevitable and serious choking incident. It did not happen. Emily swallowed the chicken without mishap and proceeded to demolish the rest of it with a beatific smile and contented cries of 'gid'.

This incident caused everyone to rethink their treatment of Emily and re-evaluate her care. With some misgivings changes were made. Emily was offered a choice of food and successfully managed to feed herself food which she could hold herself. Even if a diet of sandwiches, chips, oranges and meat was not the most balanced in the world, her meal-time tantrums disappeared.

The nurses also decided that as Emily hated her bath they would wash her at the sink instead. In spite of her incontinence this proved satisfactory. The biggest change of all, however, was when a nurse decided to try Emily in a wheelchair instead of the slightly tipped armchair in which she had spent the last three years. To everyone's amazement Emily managed to learn to manoeuvre this quite successfully by scooting it backwards with her right leg. She could move herself to the day room windows, to the table and in front of the television with few collisions.

Reflections on Emily

In Emily's story it is clear that, in spite of a sincerely 'caring' approach on the unit, the staff had failed to identify this patient's real needs. They had assumed that she was 'incompetent', and acting out that assumption actually made her less able than she would otherwise have been. In the busy round of ensuring that Emily was dry, fed and warm her attempts to communicate were somehow missed. Her expressions of frustration were put down to dementia, all her activities were decided by someone else and, as a result, her life must have been miserable.

Emily may well have had some arteriosclerotic dementia but it would have been at an early and mild stage. No one attempted to assess her aphasia to see if she could understand what was said; no one tried to make sense of her tantrums to see if there was a pattern and a reason for them; the nurses acted on an assessment that was years old and no attempt was made to re-evaluate her abilities.

How many more helpless patients are there in this type of situation?

When a life has been narrowed so drastically by illness, as in Emily's case, it is the nurse's duty to search diligently for anything that can improve the quality of that life, to help the patient regain control, and avoid doing anything which encourages helplessness and dependency.

CONTROL AND CONFORMISM

In the case of both Elsie and Emily, although the nurses assumed a strongly paternalistic stance and exerted excessive control, there is no doubt that they acted out of genuine concern. They might recognise that they had made mistakes but their actions, in their own eyes, were prompted by a wish to protect their patients from harm. However, painful as it may be to those who care for elderly people, it must be acknowledged that some practices owe nothing to kindness. In a tiring and often frustrating branch of nursing many instances of what can only be described as assault and battery occur. (The UKCC has many fully documented cases of neglect, cruelty and other forms of abuse occurring in health care institutions.)

One suspects that these cases are only the extreme end of a continuum. Elderly patients are often forced to take drugs, may have their dignity stripped from them by failing to provide privacy in which to wash or eliminate, and their freedom to move may be curtailed by the use of tables tightly screwed to chairs, the removal of walking aids and the use of cot-sides. Worse still, perhaps, patients who could possibly have achieved rehabilitation and a return to independence are often made incontinent and dependent by nurses who fail to meet their needs because it is less trouble to wash an incontinent patient than take them to the lavatory regularly.

In many of these situations it is recognised by the nurses that the care they are giving is unacceptable, but due to a shortage of staff or resources they feel they are unable to change things. Nurses who complain of such conditions are often accused of being unable to 'cope' or of being 'inefficient'. In some cases a nurse who complains may find his or her career in ruins, as in the case of the nurse Graham Pink, dismissed by Stockport Health Authority following his 'blowing the whistle' over what he regarded as inadequate standards in his care of the elderly ward.

The really worrying thing about such situations is that there are many nurses who have become used to the conditions in which poor practice prevails and, being habituated to a health care culture of unquestioning obedience, they fail to recognise that anything is wrong. In a sense, they begin to suffer from a kind of moral blindness. Let us return to the issue of falling accidents to illustrate this point.

I undertook some small-scale research into falls in a care of the elderly ward at a major London hospital in 1991.[14] I used a sample of 114 patients and 20 qualified nursing staff who cared for them. I found that the nurses usually adopted a rigidly conformist and paternalistic attitude, tending to go for control or restraint rather than more freedom for patients.

Although the nurses in my study were genuinely concerned about the trauma and distress resulting from a fall, they were not aware, and made no attempt to become aware, of the causes of falls or the best ways of preventing them. However, they were meticulous in merely reporting the falls. My questioning revealed that a significant number of the nurses would advocate preventive measures which could in fact increase the chances of dangerous falls, such as the sedation of 'at risk' patients or the use of restraining devices such as cot-sides and chairs with fixed tables.

A nurse may be perceived as quite a powerful authority figure and, indeed, supported by her institution, she does have great power over the patient. It may not even occur to elderly patients that they should complain. Sometimes they believe that to do so would result in some form of 'punishment'.

Sometimes the combination of unthinking conformist behaviour on the part of nurses and a compliant or apprehensive posture on the part of the patient can be fatal, as the following case illustrates.

The case of Mary

Mary was a patient with Parkinson's disease who had been a patient on a medical ward for seven weeks. She was admitted from home because her disease had made it increasingly difficult for her to manage. She was commenced on medication to control the tremor and a programme of physiotherapy and occupational therapy was initiated. The nursing assessment established that Mary was very constipated and a series of enemas was prescribed, together with oral laxatives. Mary continued to have problems eliminating and so the nurses continued to give an enema every three days, faithfully recording these on a 'bowel chart'.

In the seventh week of her admission during one of her regular enemas Mary suffered a perforated bowel. A severe haemorrhage occurred and Mary required surgery to repair the damage. Three days after her operation she contracted a chest infection and one week later she died.

Reflections on Mary

Mary died as a direct result of damage caused by the enemas she was given. The nurse who told this story said that the enema had become a 'habit'. The nursing team was concerned that Mary's constipation would eventually obstruct her bowel, but she did not recall any alternative methods of solving the problem. She had reflected on the incident and admitted that Mary's diet and fluid intake had not been adjusted and, when the enemas appeared to be solving the problem the doctors had not been approached to prescribe different laxatives. Even had Mary lived the administration of an enema every three days is unacceptable – it is a painful and undignified treatment. However, even in these days of 'holistic care', I would suggest that this practice is extremely common.

Mary had no relatives. No one complained or sued the hospital, so the matter was closed. Mary's nurse confessed, however, that the fear of litigation was never far from her mind.

CONCLUSION

In actual practice nurses may become blind to the denial of choices to their patients. Often they do not ask themselves the right questions. Here is an indication (and only an indication) of the kinds of questions which would pass through the mind of any conscientious nurse, one who is breaking out of the complacency of procedural routine.

Of herself:
Would I like to be in the position which the patient is being put in?
Am I being fair and impartial?
Am I being influenced by irrelevant or low priority factors (e.g. my own convenience, mere habit)?
Have I really considered all the options which could be made available to the patient?
Do I have enough knowledge about this situation to make a good decision?

Of the institution:
Is there anything I, and my colleagues, can do to improve the situation?
What are my resources and am I using them fully?
What are the policies and procedures and are they adequate?
Do I need to involve other professionals?

Of the patient:
Does the patient have a lot more potential than I think?
Is the patient being allowed sufficient freedom?
Does the patient understand?
Does the patient have adequate information?
What outside pressures are influencing the patient, such as relatives or financial matters?
What 'inner' pressures are influencing the patient, such as pain, depression, grief, or poor hearing?

Of the profession:
Do the nurses involved have sufficient power in the matter at hand, and if not how can that be rectified?
What does the Code of Conduct and similar documents have to say on this?
What are the legal implications of this particular situation?
What are the relevant moral, ethical and legal rights of the patient?

By means of case studies I have raised the issue of the elderly patient's freedom and independence. In examining the patient's freedom of choice, in the context of the health care professional's perception of risk, I have focused on the more dramatic choices such as whether a patient should go into a nursing home, take solid foods, walk around despite a high chance of falling, and be allowed to die. However, it is perhaps the little things making up the daily routine which are the real measure of the freedom and independence allowed the patient. In some hospitals even such decisions as a patient's continuing to wear a hearing aid in a noisy ward or day room or continuing to wear ill-fitting and uncomfortable dentures are made by the nursing staff.

Is the patient addressed by the name he wishes to be addressed by? Can the patient choose the nurse who cares for him? Does the patient have control over his money, and does he have the belongings with him which he wants? Does he have some control over his medication? Control over when relatives and other visitors call? Can the patient wear her own clothing, sit where she wants, choose when to go to the lavatory? Can she decide when to go to sleep and when to wake up instead of being forced into a rigid hospital regime?

The real challenge of nursing care for the elderly is that of enlarging and enhancing the freedom and control that patients have over their remaining years.

NOTES

1 The proportion of people over 65 years of age in Great Britain currently stands at just over 15 per cent. It has been estimated by demographers that, although this is a dramatic increase compared with figures at the beginning of the century (when people over 65 numbered 5 per cent of the population), it is unlikely to increase substantially. However, the proportion of very elderly people in the group will grow, with a predicted slight decline in the numbers of younger elderly people. From the health care point of view the most significant increase will be in the group aged 85 years and above because it is at this great age that people are most likely to require institutional care or intensive social services at home. As people reach their eighth decade they are more likely to suffer degenerative conditions which severely curtail mobility and cognition.
2 Townsend, P., *Poverty in the United Kingdom: A Survey of Household Resources and Standards of Living*, Harmondsworth: Penguin, 1979.
3 United Kingdom Central Council, *Code of Professional Conduct*, London: UKCC, 3rd edn, 1992.
4 Names and some details in all the cases in this chapter have been changed to preserve confidentiality. I do not intend to cast doubt on the standards at any *particular* hospital.
5 Field, P., *Attitudes Revisited: An Examination of Student Nurses' Attitudes towards Old People in Hospital*, London: Royal College of Nursing, 1986.

6 Grant, J. and Hamilton, S., 'Falls in a Rehabilitation Centre: A Retrospective and Comparative Analysis', *Rehabilitation Nursing*, 1987, vol. 12, pp. 74–7.

7 Askham, J. *et al.*, *A Review of Research on Falls Among Elderly People*, London: Age Concern Institute of Gerontology, King's College, London, 1990.

8 Redfern, S., 'The Elderly Patient', in S. Redfern (ed.), *Nursing Elderly People*, Edinburgh: Churchill Livingstone, 2nd edn, 1991, p. 551.

9 Kennedy, I., 'The Legal Effect of Requests by the Terminally Ill and Aged not to Receive Further Treatment from Doctors', *Criminal Law Review*, April 1976.

10 For a more detailed consideration of cases involving difficulties over feeding see Julie Fenton's chapter in this volume.

11 Consider the case of Dr Nigel Cox brought before Winchester Crown Court for 'attempted murder' after administering a lethal injection to his patient, a 70-year-old woman who was dying in agony and who pleaded for medical help to die. A nurse reported his action to senior nurse management. See *The Guardian*, 11 September 1992, p. 3.

12 Beauchamp, T. L. and Childress, J. F., *Principles of Biomedical Ethics*, 3rd edn, New York: Oxford University Press, 1989, p. 83.

13 I am grateful to Geoff Hunt for this point.

14 Smith, L., 'Falls Among the Elderly in an Institutional Setting: Implications for Nurse Education', unpublished M.Sc. thesis, Age Concern Institute of Gerontology, King's College, University of London, London, 1991.

Chapter 4

Caring for patients who cannot or will not eat

Julie Fenton

Many moral and ethical questions arise in relation to the feeding of patients who cannot or will not eat. How are decisions about feeding and hydration reached? What values and assumptions underlie these decisions? Is a decision not to feed or hydrate a patient always fully discussed and documented? Which courses of action are in the patient's 'best interest', and how is this 'interest' determined? How and when, if ever, should a decision not to feed or hydrate be made? Can so basic a provision as food and water ever be considered as optional care?

These questions arise in the context of modern hospitals and advanced technology. Many of our present ethical problems about feeding did not arise in the past when patients died at home and were offered sips of fluids to satiety. Often, it appears that 'technology' forces the decision whether to use a given intervention simply because it is available. Many doctors do not readily accept that it may be better to do less rather than more for a patient. Prolonging life may simply be assumed to be the overriding concern, with little thought for human dignity and the wishes of patients and families.

In modern practice there is often an underlying tension between two different understandings of 'nourishing' the patient. First, nourishing as an intrinsic part of giving care, which falls within the realm of nursing. Second, nourishing as a biological and technical process, a life-sustaining treatment under the control of the medical or nutrition team (from which the nurse may be excluded).

These situations are seldom straightforward. On the admission of a patient with a severe stroke, or one who is unconscious and unable to communicate, the decision to feed or hydrate may in fact be made by the doctor. Other members of the health care team and the family may not be consulted, or not consulted adequately. The initiation of medical treatment in an old person with a severe stroke or dementia may be seen with hindsight to be inappropriate and to represent a missed opportunity to allow dying to occur with the dignity and integrity of everyone intact. The early rescue of patients from an illness from which there is no hope of meaningful recovery may well cause distress to the patient and relatives. Nurses have a special advisory role in dealing with such situations.

A CASE STUDY

It is helpful to begin with a case. Mr Arnold was admitted to an acute ward for mentally ill elderly people, located in a large psychiatric hospital.[1] Aged 70 years, he was below the accepted age for care by psychogeriatricians, but was accepted for psychiatric assessment because the orthopaedic ward at the general hospital had been unable to provide the necessary level of care. Mr Arnold, who had no known relatives or close friends, suffered from Alzheimer's disease. He was a tall man, physically active and agitated, constantly pacing restlessly around the ward. He was also suffering from cancer of the prostate, a compound fracture of the humerus (resulting from a fall) and diabetes mellitis controllable by diet. His medication on admission was promazine and morphine.

The patient presented as extremely thin. He was tearful and complained of pain from his broken arm although he refused to wear the supporting sling. Advice from the oncologist was that no pain would be expected from his tumour at its present stage and the prognosis was for two to three years survival from the condition.

He refused most food and drink which was offered to him, taking only a few mouthfuls when pressed to do so by the nurses. He became distressed and sometimes aggressive when attempts were made to assist him at meals.

During his first three weeks of admission pain control was achieved and antidepressant medication was prescribed. However, his weight fell further, at which point the dietitian was asked to advise on his management. His energy-consuming restlessness, the tumour, fracture and his tall stature were taken into account. He was at least 10 kgs below a healthy body weight for his height. His biochemical and haematological nutritional parameters were within normal limits (other than some abnormal results related to the known pathology), with the exception of blood glucose which, despite the diabetes, was sometimes very low.

His estimated need for 3,500 kcals would be very difficult to achieve by voluntary oral intake in view of the feeding problems. The dietitian asked the ward team to consider if they wished to begin overnight nasogastric feeding, which could be employed to provide half the patient's needs whilst he slept. Ideally, the balance would be taken orally during the day. Until a consensus decision was reached, the patient was to be offered whatever was available and acceptable to him, with none of the restrictions of a 'diabetic diet'. The hypoglycaemia may have been the result of starvation, and sugar restriction had no place in his management. In addition, high protein/high energy supplementary drinks were to be offered and encouraged three times a day.

At the ward round the decision of the multidisciplinary team was that Mr Arnold would not tolerate a nasogastric tube and would be distressed by any attempt to pass one. Nevertheless, the pivot of his care was now feeding, as a continuing weight loss would soon prove fatal. Representatives of all disciplines were able to contribute to the discussion at the ward round, but it was the decision of the nursing staff that they would somehow find a way to stop this patient from wasting away before their eyes. A nutritional plan to meet the patient's needs was devised by the dietitian and nurses together. The nurses agreed to encourage, persuade and even cajole the patient to take a supplement nine times a day in addition to his meals.

Although Mr Arnold liked the taste of his 'special drinks', he remained extremely reluctant to drink or eat. For most of the day a nurse was to be seen at his side urging him to 'take a little more', so that one drink would be finished before the next one was due. Soon he was spending most of the day seated quietly in the nursing office, alongside the desk upon which he rested a glass of nourishment which he was slowly imbibing. The treatment was effective, not only in improving his intake but in stopping his restless pacing around the ward. He gained 0.7 kg in the first week and this encouraged everyone to persevere. Slowly his appetite improved, and his mental state improved too within the limits of his dementia. As he took more of the ward food the number of supplements was adjusted downwards until he was taking only two or three a day. The improvement in his weight and physical and mental health was sustained for two months.

However, the fractured arm deteriorated as he still refused to co-operate in keeping it still. He once again became more resistant to the gentle but persistent pressure from the nurses to eat and drink and started to lose weight again.

It had proved impossible to find a suitable nursing home to which Mr Arnold could be discharged, and when a bed became available on a continuing care ward within the psychiatric hospital he was transferred there. The prescription for nutritional support was renewed by the dietitian on the new ward and the nurses agreed to be as encouraging as possible. However, it appears that nutrition was no longer the highest priority in his care, and weight loss continued. Mr Arnold died within six weeks of the transfer.

TO FEED OR NOT

Tube-feeding

Nasogastric feeding may, under some clinical circumstances, be used to feed patients. Modern fine-bore tubes and pumps which ensure controlled delivery of the feed, together with manufactured feeds designed to meet a wide variety of metabolic and absorptive conditions, have eliminated many of the common complications and distress associated with tube-feeding in the past. Such advances still have not completely eliminated fears and anxieties about 'force-feeding'. To the patient the use of nasogastric tubes may be seen as an assault or an invasion rather than as a form of medical treatment or nourishment.

The distress and upset which may be caused to the patient by tube-feeding should not be dismissed, and was taken into account in Mr Arnold's case. In the alert patient it entails the loss of control over the choice of food and timing of meals. The very presence of the tube is a visible sign of a loss of appetite and an underlying pathology, and this has its impact on the patient's self-image. Furthermore, the long-term use of nasogastric feeding necessitates regular blood tests to check that the patient's biochemistry and haematology are satisfactory. Given the risks, tube-feeding ethically requires that the patient be monitored. But the long-term benefits to a dying person of the blood tests may be in doubt.

Where possible, nursing care should encourage patients to express their feelings about tube-feeding. If such feelings become too painful then artificial feeding may be rejected. A difficult ethical issue is under what conditions the patient may exercise the right to reject such feeding. If restraint is needed to prevent the patient from removing a feeding tube, then nutrition is being maintained at what may be an ethically unacceptable cost. Patient comfort and acceptance may well be the deciding factor in the administration of hydration and nutrition by artificial means.

On the other hand, the availability of the necessary support and resources may be a constraint and it could be argued that this situation is an injustice to the patient who needs and wants the nutritional support. Some other methods of artificial feeding require intensive resourcing, but I will not discuss these here.[2]

Withholding nutrition

Unless the condition has been the result of inanition or dehydration, feeding and hydration does not cure or improve a terminal state, but will sustain biological life so that other treatments can be given. Feeding may in some circumstances prolong the process of dying and may cause avoidable suffering to the dying patient.

One might take the view that it is often morally right to withhold nutrition from a dying patient. I will not discuss the legal aspects of this. Generally speaking, as Young has written:

> The law accepts that there is no point in prolonging the life of some patients when treatment has no useful purpose. The patient whose death is imminent most definitely falls into this category. It is then quite legal to omit care, even when that omission will allow the patient to die.[3]

It is generally regarded as ethically permissible to withhold treatment which would serve mainly to prolong the dying process. Mr Arnold, we recall, had a prognosis of about three years of life and the question of withholding feeding did not arise. In the case of an elderly dying patient, for example, there may be a strong argument for regarding the withholding of nutrition and hydration administered by vein or gastric tube as not only morally permissible but morally required. Continuing with feeding may cause suffering or prolong it. Some would take the view that, if needed for comfort, spoon-feeding may be continued.

All the same, one has to recognise that some people, often taking a strongly religious position, would object on moral grounds to the withholding or withdrawal of food and/or fluids under any, or any but the most extreme, circumstances. In what follows I am thinking mainly of people who do not take such a view, but who may still feel confused or unhappy about withholding or withdrawal.

As one might expect, the withdrawal of nutrition may evoke profound emotional responses in the health care staff and the family of the patient.[4] The emotional and moral significance of giving food and fluids is generally different from that of interventions such as giving an injection or an enema. In fact, it is curious perhaps to speak of giving food and fluids as 'intervention' at all. For example, when an uncomfortable treatment is given to a conscious but dying patient who cannot benefit from the treatment, this often arouses feelings of futility in the nurse. But the cessation of intravenous fluids or enteral nutrition may be experienced by the nurse who removes the apparatus as an act of 'euthanasia' or even 'murder' – although she may not openly express it in these terms. If she does not experience this, she may be afraid that others who do will condemn her for indifference.

Given what she feels is expected of her as a nurse, she may not be able to see, or may be unable to accept her better judgement, that withholding feeding/hydration may be the right thing to do, and she may try to live with the feeling of futility instead. Such a reaction on the part of the nurse may also be evident when the patient is unconscious and will never recover consciousness. It may be difficult to accept withholding or withdrawal of treatment, even when the treatment is of no real benefit and sometimes even when it is clearly not wanted by the patient.

The decision to withhold or withdraw nutrition should always be made very carefully and involve discussion with the patient and/or the relatives and significant others as well as the health care team. The decision should be guided by several factors.

First, knowledge of the patient's own desires and values, to the extent to which they were expressed before the patient became unable to express a view.

Second, if the patient's own desires cannot be ascertained there is a duty to act in his or her best interests – which will include the relief of suffering, the preservation or restoration of functioning, the quality as well as the extent of life, and the impact of the decision on those closest to the patient.[5]

Third, if there is any doubt as to prognosis, then medical expertise should be consulted or reconsulted. Of course, accurate prognosis does not in itself resolve all the moral problems, but to deal with personal and professional doubts and tensions the nurse also needs knowledge about the medical and physiological processes involved in dying and the role of nutrition and fluids. On the basis of this knowledge, she may come to be less certain that feeding and hydration are always right.

Nearly everyone would agree that the final decision on whether to withhold/withdraw medical hydration or nutrition in the terminally ill patient needs to be made on an individual basis with paramount importance attached to relief of the patient's distress. The nurse may come to see that easing a patient's death is very often an act of nursing care.

The character of the ethical issue of feeding and hydration usually depends to some extent on the degree of understanding and choice that the patient is able to exercise. Some elderly patients with permanent mild impairment of understanding have been described as 'pleasantly senile'. They may be limited in their abilities to initiate activities and communicate but appear to be enjoying their lives. Freedom from discomfort should be the overriding objective in their care, and withholding feeding is not usually an issue at all. Ethically, a more difficult situation for the nurse is the severely and irreversibly demented patient who does not initiate purposeful activity but may accept food with complete passivity or violently refuse nourishment and bodily care. There may be no easy answer in such cases, but multidisciplinary discussion and the involvement of relatives is nearly always helpful.

In the extreme case of a patient in whom brain death has been confirmed or one in a persistent vegetative state (perhaps the neocortex is largely and irreversibly destroyed, although some brain-stem functions persist), it is usually considered ethically justified to withhold treatment such as antibiotics, hydration and nutrition, allowing the patient to die. However, even here some might take the view that life is absolutely sacred and that feeding and hydration should continue as far as possible.

Fluids

One may consider the question of hydration separately from that of feeding in so far as a decision not to feed does not entail a decision not to hydrate. Situations arise in which a patient is not being fed and is still being hydrated.

If the decision is made to give fluids by intravenous route, one should ask what the beneficial effects of hydration are likely to be?

The patient may be less nauseated and may experience an increased alertness and sense of well-being as electrolyte levels are normalised. A fluid deficit, and reduced circulation in all body systems, may cause electrolyte concentration and acidosis, nausea and vomiting. Uraemia may cause neuromuscular irritability with twitching and restlessness and a progressively lower level of consciousness. There are other discomforts, which may, however, be treated or ameliorated.[6]

Nutritionally, intravenous fluids are not a source of food to the patient. Often the outcome of spoon-feeding or intravenous fluids is delayed death due to slow starvation or an intervening infection.

Zerwekh, writing on the care of the dying cancer patient, asks, 'Is it more merciful to give the dying patient fluids than to let him experience dehydration?'[7] Indeed, it is not obvious that giving fluids is always the right thing to do. There is a need for more discussion of whether dehydration causes or alleviates suffering. It might be argued that for the patient for whom death is imminent and inevitable dehydration may ease death. It may add to the patient's comfort and peace during the final stages of life, allowing a dignified death.[8] Hydration may cause acute discomfort to the patient near death. It may be necessary to pass a urinary catheter if the kidneys are functioning. If the kidneys have shut down, as is common before death, the extra fluids cannot be excreted and accumulate in the body tissues. It may become necessary to aspirate the stomach contents. An increase in pulmonary secretions may require suction to be applied. An increase in oedema may cause an increase in pain for the patient with a tumour.

A compromise solution may sometimes be considered the best. For example, a reduced volume of intravenous fluids may give some benefit in terms of well-being without causing problems such as those mentioned above.

Nurses have sometimes found it very difficult to accept that reducing or stopping hydration could be the humane and proper thing to do, but this is generally because they have not had full knowledge of the physiological facts.

DECISION MAKING AND THE NURSE

Double-binds and distance

In some cases a medical decision not to use tube-feeding and intravenous fluids is made, resulting in a difficult nursing decision about whether to persist with spoon-feeding or not. Not to spoon-feed may be seen as allowing the patient to die. Nurses may be uncertain as to what is the most merciful decision. They may not be sure what is happening to the patient and what their responsibility for the patient's condition is. Is the patient dying from dehydration? Is the thirst making her suffer? Is it causing her pain?

Not unsurprisingly, carers feel that they cause suffering when the patient, unable to say how she feels, reacts as though food hurts her stomach when swallowed. The patient may frequently swallow the wrong way, almost choking. Sometimes the patient shows panic when fed. Nurses may feel that whatever they do they will be doing the wrong thing. This is one kind of double-bind in which the nurse feels trapped and unable to resolve the conflict.

The nurse who will be carrying out the medical decision to feed or not to feed may not have been offered the opportunity to voice her opinion. She often encounters an ethical and professional dilemma: the nurse is deemed responsible for the activity of nursing care and thus for withholding any nursing activity but is not allowed to exercise that responsibility, or must exercise it in partial ignorance. When things go wrong she may be held responsible even though she was at the time in question not expected or encouraged to understand or question. If she questions she may be in trouble, and if she does not question she is in trouble – here is another double-bind.

For example, an order to 'encourage oral intake' when the patient no longer eats often leaves the nurse in an impossible position. She may respond by losing sensitivity to the needs and feelings of the patient, who then becomes a victim of impersonal care.

In this situation it is not surprising if the patient comes to distrust the care worker, and may exhibit this in various forms of protest such as rejecting food. This may lead to the use of force which in turn leads to greater distrust and more protest. The patient may feel humiliated and indulge in spitting and spilling which in turn humiliate the care worker. The carer blames the patient and the patient punishes the nurse. Spitting, 'playing' with food and 'fighting' against the care worker may be an attempt to communicate when the ability to speak is lost.

Norberg and colleagues have considered the effect of the double-bind experienced by nurses responsible for feeding patients with advanced dementia who are refusing food or fluids.[9] They claim that it results in the nurse distancing from the patient and in scapegoating amongst the carers.

In situations where workers are not allowed to discuss the issues of death and suffering, so that eventually they may not even allow themselves to think about them, there are very detrimental consequences for the standards of care. The defence mechanism of distancing leads to care that is cold, mechanical and without understanding. The final outcome may be sadism – the carer hurts the patient physically or psychologically as a defence against her own guilt and anxiety.

In scapegoating the emphasis is on blaming another person for giving an order which is morally difficult or unacceptable. The carer can then concentrate on the character of the person who gave the order rather than on the patient and improving the situation. The consequences of these dynamics are serious for staff co-operation and thus serious for patients. The person who gives the order, perhaps the ward doctor or dietitian, may turn away or flee which usually lead to even more blame, so a vicious circle is perpetuated.[10]

Multidisciplinary approach

Adequate staffing and resources, patience and the effort to understand the patient's needs, as well as skills, such as a good spoon-feeding technique, are clearly essential. But in many ways what is most needed is open discussion and co-operation. It is often the nurse who alerts the doctor to the fact that spoon-feeding and drinking are failing, but she may have little or no input in the decisions which follow. In the worst scenario if the doctor decides without discussion to tube-feed, he may be condemned as the tormentor of the patient, and if he decides not to tube-feed he may be regarded as a 'murderer'.

Doctors and nurses need to explore each others' assumptions and values to understand better the basis of their disagreements and underlying tensions over the treatment and care undertaken or proposed. If 'being alive' is always valued higher than health, and the length of life is thought more important than its quality, then it is easy to justify the decision to tube-feed. Important factors influencing nursing decisions about food are the patient's viewpoint, the patient's comfort and peace of mind, the 'symbolic' significance of food and fluids in nurturing and caring, and the role of the patient's relatives and friends.

The role of the nurse needs to be better understood, not only by medical and paramedical staff but by nurses themselves. The responsibility for feeding and hydration as part of nursing care necessitates the full participation of the nurse in the decision making and an understanding of the reasoning behind the decisions made. Studies have shown that nurses often stress the need for sufficient information on which to base a decision.[11]

Gallagher-Allred states that the nursing goals of nutritional care are to maximise the enjoyment of life and to minimise pain.[12] If eating is not an enjoyable experience it should not be emphasised. The nurse can be a strong patient advocate and family ally by reassuring both that loving care can be demonstrated in ways other than through feeding.

The nurse's role also involves assessing whether some modifications in diet can alleviate symptoms and improve well-being. It is important to identify the family's and patient's nutritional concerns and to integrate nutritional goals into the overall care plan.

The level of care appropriate for the stage of the disease process should be designated, and multidisciplinary decisions should be taken (as in the case of Mr Arnold), carefully documented and all personnel need to be aware of them and adhere to them. Anorexia and cachexia are hallmark conditions of many end-stage chronic diseases. This is particularly true for patients with incurable cancer, renal disease, pulmonary disease, AIDS and heart failure. Terminal illness may lead to changes in the need for nutrients and to malabsorption related either to the primary disease or to the treatment itself. The dying process slows many bodily functions including gastric emptying which may lead to anorexia.

Anger, grief and depression may all lead to food refusal. Appetite may return as these feelings are resolved. The nurse needs to know whether food or fluid refusal are perceived as a problem by patient, the family or both. The patient can be freed from the pressure to eat when attention is shifted from maintaining the patient's nutritional status to enhancing patient comfort by other means, which may include providing small appetizing meals. Sometimes it is better to offer no food unless the patient requests it.

PATHOLOGY AND VALUES

Is feeding 'treatment'?

Feeding and giving fluids may not be regarded as 'medical treatment' at all, but as so fundamental that one could not ever deny them to anyone. Dresser asks, 'Ought we to regard tube and intravenous feeding as forms of medical treatment, or should we classify them with more basic sorts of care?'[13] If we necessarily associate feeding with respect and care for a dying person we may be less willing to stop feeding than to stop medical treatment.

Is the provision of food and fluid a treatment or intervention in the same sense as, for example, a transfusion of blood, with which it has much biochemically in common. Many patients in long-stay geriatric care are not immediately close to death, until they refuse or are unable to take food or fluids. It has been observed that, 'Food and water are so central to an array of human emotions that it is almost impossible to consider them with the same emotional detachment that one might feel toward a respirator or a dialysis machine.'[14] Doctors perhaps are inclined to see feeding and giving water as 'nutrition' and 'hydration', and apply standard medical criteria in making a decision, whereas nurses (like the relatives) are more inclined to see nutrition and hydration as 'feeding' and 'giving a drink' and make decisions in more 'personal' terms.

There may also be a temptation to ascribe any refusal to eat directly to pathology. Cognisant of a general duty to keep patients alive, some carers see the patient's not eating as a consequence of brain dysfunction, not as a lack of desire or a willingness to die. Nurses who see the matter this way are more prepared to use a considerable amount of force and usually do not experience anxiety about this.

If nutritional supports are to be withheld or withdrawn the nurse should ensure that the entire health care team is aware of the 'symbolic' or 'moral' meaning of this step. But while there is a danger in conceiving the question in 'purely clinical' terms, there is also a danger in ignoring the physiological facts. The provision of food and water is so important that family, friends and staff need to have someone put to them that many patients in a terminal situation are not aware of hunger or thirst and that trying to satisfy a supposed hunger or thirst may cause or prolong suffering.

The culture and environment of eating

There are many causes of refusal/inability to eat, not least of which sometimes is simply the fact of being in an institution. Being taken out of one's home and one's chosen routine of meal times, and losing the control one has over what one eats, is usually disturbing. To fail to understand this elementary fact may lead to unethical and paternalistic behaviour on the part of nurses and other health carers.

One should also consider the possibility of mental health problems, socio-cultural problems, medication side-effects, staff attitudes or actions, the decline in sensory enjoyment of food which is normally associated with ageing, uncomfortable dentures or sore mouth, the fear of death, and the quality, quantity, appearance or manner of presentation of the food. Environmental odours either from urine, disinfectants or room fresheners and deodorants, to which the nurse may have become used, may (obviously) cause loss of appetite.

Eating may provide an opportunity for the person to express an independence and control which they cannot exert in other aspects of their lives in an institution. They may complain about food even when it is good because they are unable to complain about abuse, feelings of worthlessness, loneliness or frustration. A patient may reject food to punish a member of staff who has been unkind. Food may be spat out, spilled or played with as a form of revenge or non-cooperation. Eating 'problems' may be a means of calling attention to unanswered needs.

Pre-admission and admission care plans should include an acknowledgement of the personal, cultural and religious aspects of food. Lifelong food habits may be vital in ensuring the acceptability of institutional food. It should be obvious that food which does not conform to cultural patterns will not be considered good or nourishing. A patient may even feel humiliated by having to eat certain kinds of food.

A respect for privacy and 'territory' may be important at meals, especially for the older person, more so when the patient is embarrassed by his difficulties in eating. Habits, and rituals of order, decorum and cleanliness at meals, are important for people of all ages and if these are ignored the person may not eat well or not at all. One should not need to point out that the social niceties surrounding eating maintain the sense of personal worth and esteem.

The separation of people with differing degrees of eating difficulties and different standards may be helpful, as one person may put another 'off' his food. Some people with physical problems in eating but with normal awareness may prefer to be alone to eat if they feel self-conscious. Some patients may not eat because they fear choking. This cause of food refusal may be ameliorated by choice of suitable food textures and feeding techniques.

A patients' council, with real influence on the menu and the eating routine, is usually a worthwhile initiative. Attractive separate dining rooms and seating arrangements should be arranged and personal events such as birthdays celebrated. Most patients are grateful for menus in large print, having someone ensure that their spectacles are clean and hearing aids are worn and turned on. Problems of mouth health and denture fit may easily be overlooked on the assumption that the refusal of food is pathologically caused.

Silent suicide

Simon uses the term 'silent suicide' to describe elderly bed-ridden patients who have apparently decided to end their lives by passively refusing food or fluid.[15] Such patients, who may be regarded as competent and for whom death is not imminent, must be distinguished from terminally ill patients for whom death is imminent and who refuse further treatment in order not to prolong dying.

Persons refusing to eat or comply with medication may do so without warning or drawing attention to their true motives. Silent suicide may therefore be unrecognised. Family members may veto intervention on the grounds that further suffering would result. When an elderly person, who appears to have no underlying pathology causing food refusal, rejects medication and stops eating and drinking, then one is morally obliged, I believe, to explore the possibility of covert depression. Treatment for depression can sometimes bring a remarkable change in the patient. Admittedly, 'depression' is not always an easy diagnosis to make. If one is satisfied that the patient is not depressed then intervention may be wrong. There is always the possibility that 'silent suicide' may be a perfectly rational decision rather than a sign of depression.

Factors precipitating depression in elderly people include physical illness, loss of an important relationship, institutional living, loss of independence, loss of financial resources, loss of occupational identity, a co-existing psychiatric disorder, drugs, alcohol, physical or emotional abuse, and a genetic-biological vulnerability to depression. It is critically important to refrain from jumping to conclusions which might have crucial moral implications. For example, if it turns out that an elderly patient is depressed it does not follow that he is 'incompetent' and that all decisions should be arrogated to the health care professional. At the same time one should not see 'depression' in every act of refusal.

CONCLUSION

Nutritional support is not to be given unthinkingly, without moral and ethical sensitivity. For some patients continued nourishment is more burdensome than beneficial. The challenge is to make sure that it is only in respect of such patients that non-feeding is approved. As patients' advocates, who are (or should be) close to patients and responsible for their care, nurses have a strong duty to ensure that an informed and balanced decision is made about food and water.

Unfortunately, the ethical and legal concerns of nurses are often ignored. Open discussion and a broader understanding of the ethical issues involved are necessary for the good of the patient and the care staff, and would reduce interpersonal and interprofessional tensions. Nurses need not be powerless, complying with orders they feel are morally unjustified. They have a responsibility to open the ethical dialogue concerning what is an appropriate level of care for a terminally ill patient unable to express his wishes.

NOTES

1   I am grateful to Geoff Hunt for his assistance in reworking this chapter, and to Frances O'Brien who collaborated with me on an earlier brief article. In the case study the name and identifying details have been changed.
2   In enterostomy feeding the feeding tube is surgically introduced directly into the stomach or duodenum through the wall of the abdomen. Bolus feeding, rather than continuous drip feeding, has the advantage that the patient is not attached to a feeding pump and has mobility and independence. A functioning digestive tract is essential for both methods of enteral feeding and they are not normally undertaken unless the advice of a dietitian or specialist nurse is available for support. When the gastro-intestinal tract is non-functioning, nutritional intake may be maintained by means of total parenteral nutrition through either a peripheral or central vein. The resource commitment and clinical

management for long-term use are often problematic with thrombosis and infections common side-effects. In some centres treating AIDS patients, the request for such support has come from patients and the ethical issues of equity in the use of resources has become an issue.

3 Young, A., *Law and Professional Conduct in Nursing*, London: Scutari, 1991, p. 71. Some guidance on legal aspects of feeding may also be found in Kennedy, I. and Grubb, A., *Medical Law: Text and Materials*, London: Butterworth, 1989, ch. 14. See also Ann Young's chapter in this volume, especially her discussion of patients unable to give consent.

4 Printz, L. A., 'Is Withholding Hydration a Valid Comfort Measure?', *Geriatrics*, 1988, vol. 43 (11), pp. 84–8.

5 See Creighton, H., 'Decisions on Food and Fluid in Life Sustaining Measures', *Nursing Management*, 1984, vol. 15 (6), pp. 47–9 and vol. 15 (7), pp. 54–6.

6 Dry mouth with cracking of the mucosa and inflammation may be painful, food debris and dried sputum may coat the mouth. The mouth may be subject to infections, especially thrush. Good nursing care of oral hygiene and the use of ice chips and small sips of oral fluids, coating the lips with a protective moisturising preparation, in addition to local anaesthetic and drug therapy for infections will relieve discomfort from these causes.

7 Zerwekh, J. V., 'The Dehydration Question', *Nursing*, 1983, vol. 83 (13), pp..47–51.

8 A disorder in thirst perception may protect the patient from discomfort. Also, dehydration means that there is a decreased urine output, fewer bouts of vomiting, reduced pulmonary secretions with less coughing, less pharyngeal secretions so that dysphagia, choking and drowning become less of a problem. Peripheral and pulmonary oedema is reduced resulting in reduction in pressure around tumours, which often leads to a decrease in the need for painkillers. The increased electrolytes have a natural anaesthetic effect on the central nervous system resulting in a lower level of consciousness and lower perception of suffering. On how dehydration may ease death see Watts, D. T. and Cassel, C. K., 'Extraordinary Nutritional Support: A Case Study and Ethical Analysis', *Journal of the American Geriatrics Society*, 1984, vol. 32 (3), pp. 237–42.

9 Norberg, A., Norberg, B. and Bexell, G., 'Ethical Problems in Feeding Patients with Advanced Dementia', *British Medical Journal*, 1980, vol. 281, pp. 847–8. Also useful are: Norberg, A., Norberg, B., Gippert, H. and Bexell, G., 'Ethical Conflicts in Long-term Care of the Aged: Nutritional Problems and the Patient–care Worker Relationship', *British Medical Journal*, 1980, vol. 280, pp. 377–8; Norberg, A., Asplund, K. and Waxman, H., 'Withdrawing Feeding and Withholding Artificial Nutrition from Severely Demented Patients. Interviews with Caregivers', *Western Journal of Nursing Research*, 1987, vol. 9 (3), pp. 348–56.

10 Athlin, E. and Norberg, A., 'Care-givers' Attitudes to and Interpretations of the Behaviour of Severely Demented Patients During Feeding

in a Patient Assignment Care System', *International Journal of Nursing Studies*, 1987, vol. 24 (2), pp. 145–53.

11 Davidson and his colleagues looked at nursing attitudes in eight different countries among nurses caring for terminally ill cancer patients and found that nurses claim they have insufficient information. See Davidson, B., Vander Laan, R., Hirschfeld, M., Norberg, A., Pitman, E. and Ju Ying, L., 'Ethical Reasoning Associated with the Feeding of Terminally Ill Cancer Patients. An International Perspective', *Cancer Nursing*, 1990, vol. 13 (5), pp. 286–92.

12 Gallagher-Allred, C. R., 'Nutritional Care of the Terminally Ill Patient and Family', in J. Penson and R. Fisher (eds), *Palliative Care for People with Cancer*, London: Edward Arnold, 1989, ch. 6, pp. 91–104.

13 Dresser, R., 'When Patients Resist Feeding: Medical, Ethical and Legal Considerations', *Journal of the American Geriatrics Society*, 1985, vol. 33 (11), pp. 790–4. This quotation is from p. 790.

14 Lynn, J. and Childress, J. F., 'Must Patients Always Be Given Food and Water?', *Hastings Center Report*, 1983, vol. 13 (17); quoted in Dresser, op. cit., p. 790. Consider too the case of Tony Bland, a football fan who suffered severe brain damage in the Hillsborough disaster and fell into a permanent vegetative state. Controversy centred on whether the discontinuation of artificial feeding would bring a charge of murder partly on the ground that feeding is not treatment. See *The Guardian*, editorial, 16 September 1992. A court finally ruled that artificial feeding could be withdrawn and Bland allowed to die. Pro-life demonstrations followed the decision. See Melanie Phillips' commentary in *The Guardian*, 5 February 1993 and Dr J. G. Howe's response in a letter in the same newspaper dated 10 February 1993.

15 Simon, R., 'Silent Suicide in the Elderly', *Bulletin of the American Academy of Psychiatry*, 1989, vol. 17 (1), pp. 83–95.

Chapter 5

Disabled people and the ethics of nursing research

Maddie Blackburn

INTRODUCTION

Aims

This chapter does not intend to present survey results or discuss their implications for service provision. I seek to discuss the ethics of undertaking nursing research, particularly of a sensitive nature, namely that involving the co-operation of disabled people, some of whom may have cognitive or learning difficulties, and may be disadvantaged and demeaned by peers. Doctors and nurses often administer treatments underestimating the disabled client's abilities and vulnerability. I address and discuss some of the ethical considerations which arose during the course of my own research. It was during this research that I came to see such considerations to be as integral and important as the research 'method' and 'results'.

I shall consider some of the moral responsibilities of a nurse researcher – particularly one working in a multidisciplinary team, contractually accountable to both a funding body (a charity) and a medical faculty, but professionally accountable to her own professional body, the United Kingdom Central Council for Nursing, Midwifery and Health Visiting (UKCC). I suggest some ways of handling the ethical questions which arise. I hope to encourage nurse researchers to think and argue more critically and with greater ethical awareness.

A primary ethical problem for researchers working with people with disabilities is that while they may appear able to give informed consent (and one should never presuppose that they cannot) their comprehension is in some cases questionable. At the same time excluding people with disabilities from research may do them a disservice by failing to obtain potential nursing knowledge.[1] I shall discuss ethical aspects of my sexuality studies related to spina bifida and hydrocephalus. I appreciate that the views and experiences are in some respects personal and do not necessarily represent those of other research nurses.

Spina bifida and hydrocephalus

In order to understand some of the dilemmas encountered through the course of my own research, it is necessary to offer some description of neural tube defects and their associated difficulties, before addressing the ethics of undertaking sexuality research.

There are several forms of spina bifida. The term literally means split spine; occulta, myelomeningocoele and meningocoele being the most common types. The neural tube in spina bifida fails to develop properly and becomes bifid. The split may occur in any part of the vertebral column but is usually just above or below waist level. The physical complications associated with this condition will vary considerably depending on the level of the spinal lesion affected and the extent of nerve damage to the spinal cord. Often paralysis below the waist and continence difficulties are associated with this condition. Some people may have some sexual dysfunction because of nerve damage to the sexual nerves running to the genitalia.[2] Although the number of children born with spina bifida has declined significantly in the last two decades, the number with this condition surviving into adulthood and requiring access to services and information has significantly increased as a result of advances in medical treatment.

Hydrocephalus is the accumulation and imbalance of the production and drainage of cerebro-spinal fluid (CSF) into the circulation. CSF is produced continuously within the four ventricles of the brain. Normally CSF passes through the intraventricular spaces, into the brain and down the spinal cord. If the drainage pathways are occluded fluid will accumulate in the ventricles, causing swelling and compression of the surrounding tissues and the baby's head will enlarge. The problems associated with this condition are complex and varied. These may include specific learning difficulties, a lack of innate intellectual ability and defective immediate and retentive memory, sequencing difficulties and poor attention span. Hydrocephalus frequently accompanies open spina bifida.

Of those participating in our studies, approximately 91 per cent of the spina bifida sample had hydrocephalus.[3] Although spina bifida and hydrocephalus are frequently described and discussed in the literature together the complications of each disability are individual and complex. Hydrocephalus may arise both from acquired and congenital causes. Spina bifida is a congenital condition. Birth prevalence for both these conditions varies in different parts of the world.[4]

SEXUALITY RESEARCH

For many years the subject of sexuality, particularly that of disabled people, has been regarded by many as taboo. Some people may have difficulty relating to their own sexuality, let alone discussing the subject with others. Our society has only recently begun to accept that sexuality should be rationally discussed and have a place in the curriculum.[5] People with physical disabilities and learning difficulties have the same interests in, and many of the same concerns about, sexuality as their able-bodied peers. They therefore have the same rights and require the same access to appropriate sexuality information acceptable to their cultural, religious, moral norms as able-bodied people.[6]

Sexuality literature suggests that sexual knowledge about and education of neurologically disabled teenagers are limited.[7] Teaching and materials require adequate planning and considered instruction, carefully designed to suit the individual's cognitive ability. In attempting to design curriculum content, does the researcher have the right to ask disabled people about their sexual history and experiences? One might ask, what research has been carried out on *able-bodied* young adults and was it ethical?

One investigative sexuality study involving the co-operation of able-bodied adults was Masters and Johnson's 1966 empirical study of human sexual response. Initially they invited the participation of prostitutes. When the researchers subsequently excluded most of the 'prostitute' data from their results, it was not because they came to think they were selecting individuals who might already be considered exploited and demeaned by society. Rather it was because of their 'migratory tendencies' and the 'varying degrees of pathology of the reproductive organs usually present in this population, precluding the possibility of establishing a secure baseline of anatomic normalcy'.[8] Yet despite having to reconsider the appropriateness of their research sample these researchers were not deterred from continuing their studies.

Is there a need for sexuality research in relation to disability? People with disabilities, who are incontinent or confined to a wheelchair, have particular and realistic concerns about forming and maintaining relationships, both with their able-bodied and disabled peers. As one might expect, the self-awareness and sexual interest of people with disabilities often increases during adolescence, albeit often in their late teens. It is now recognised that some sexuality research provides limited results. Investigative, but non-prescriptive research might arguably be considered unethical if no recommendations are provided as a result.

In 1990 the Association for Spina Bifida and Hydrocephalus (ASBAH) established a nationwide counselling service in response to a growing number of enquiries from young adults, parents and carers, for information regarding sexuality and disability. Information and advice about sex education, relationships, marriage, continence, genetic risks and love-making were the major focus of these enquiries. It became clear that there was a paucity of available information and educational material suitable for this client group, and ASBAH financed a study of the 'sexual knowledge and experiences of young adults with spina bifida and/or hydrocephalus'. 'Young adults' were those in the 16- to 25-year-old range.

It was hoped that the knowledge gained would lead to the production of useful materials, as well as offering preliminary evaluation of the efficacy of the charity's newly established counselling service. The study is now complete, some pilot training materials have been produced and evaluated and (at the time of writing) further materials are being developed. Regrettably, financial pressure forced the closure of the charity's counselling service prior to the study's completion, making its evaluation impossible. Although evaluation of the counselling service was a secondary aim of the study, I felt disappointed that I was unable to use the survey results to make any proposals for the counselling service's development particularly on issues related to sexuality.

EXERCISING ACCOUNTABILITY IN RESEARCH

Nurse researchers, like clinical nurses, are often required to bring a variety of skills to their work. They require good negotiation and communication skills not only in order to work competently and confidently with research subjects and their families but also with members of ethics committees, medical and paramedical colleagues, and other agencies.

Depending on the nature of the investigation, there may be a conflict between the nurse's respect for the pursuit and advancement of scientific knowledge and concerns about whether investigation and or assessment are in the client's considered best interest. Nurses are often required to assist doctors with the execution of research, often administering prescribed drugs or treatments on their behalf. The drugs intended, for example, as a cancer treatment may be given as part of a clinical trial, but the nurses may worry about possible iatrogenesis (medically induced complications). The nurse may question her own role and responsibilities when asked to administer treatments or medications to patients which she may feel should have been administered by the doctor.

As a nurse researcher, my primary task is to collect, analyse, prepare and disseminate information and data in a form acceptable to both the client and the funding/employing body. It happens that my current research supervisor is a doctor of medicine. Although we firmly acknowledge and respect each others' professional boundaries, I am aware that there are certain tasks which, if undertaken by me, would breach my professional code of practice. On such occasions it is my responsibility to maintain the boundaries and seek the assistance of others more qualified to perform these tasks.

In terms of professional ethics, the research nurse who may find such decisions difficult, should consider clause four of the UKCC's Code of Professional Conduct.[9] It states that you, the nurse, should acknowledge 'any limitations in your knowledge and competence and decline any duties or responsibilities unless able to perform them in a safe and skilled manner'. At the same time, clause six reminds you to 'work in a collaborative and co-operative manner with health care professionals and others involved in providing care, and recognise and respect their particular contributions within the team'.

One should never lose sight of the fact that ultimately health care research is about bringing benefits to people. Some research (therapeutic research) obviously aims to be of direct benefit to the research subject. In other kinds of research (non-therapeutic) the aim is to advance scientific knowledge, but here too it should be envisaged as benefiting a client group as a whole, even if it is not expected to give direct benefit to the research subjects. There are ethical and legal difficulties here which I shall come to later.

CONSENT

Competence and self-advocacy

There is a pressing need to ensure that clients, particularly people with physical disabilities and learning difficulties, fully comprehend the nature, extent and time of their expected involvement in a research programme. People with disabilities should not be coerced into participation by researchers. The primary interest of some researchers may be professional development or securing suitable programmes of study in which to obtain a higher qualification.

Competency to consent may be regarded in terms of three integral components: free choice, knowledge and understanding, and competency to decide.[10] Some people with learning difficulties are often capable of making decisions about daily care but may have difficulty in understanding details about operations, treatments and research involvement. Total incompetence should never be presupposed, and is only found in the profoundly mentally handicapped person. Gunn points out 'that there is no legal decision that a person who is mentally handicapped is necessarily incapable of making treatment or care decisions'.[11] It has to be admitted that 'competence' is itself a rather vague concept. Measures of competence may vary according to the institution where the research is being undertaken. Some institutions use psychological testing, others use educational attainment as indicators of cognitive function.

How often do we allocate decision making to carers or relatives with a certain disregard for the individual feelings, contributions and expectations of disabled people themselves?

Consider, for example, attitudes involved in admission and discharge from hospital, respite care, or returning to the community after a particular institution is closed. The disabled person is often allowed little choice in the decisions affecting him or her. Admittedly, this situation may arise not so much from the attitude of individual carers as from a bureaucracy which, for instance, orders the closure of a particular institution with little consultation. In fact, some carers are frequently over-protective about the disabled person taking important decisions alone. Where there is genuine concern, surely the disabled person has a right and should be encouraged to share and choose in the decision making process.

Times are changing, and self-advocacy is increasing among people with disabilities. Choice, based on explanation, is increasingly coming to be seen as a basic human right, whether it is about the freedom and independence to refuse to participate in a research project or the choice to wear one's own clothes in hospital. One cannot over-emphasize that the disabled person has the same right to explanation of the research protocol as the able-bodied do. A preliminary, coherent explanation of research objectives should always be offered by an independent, impartial interviewer in addition to sending a coherent, explanatory letter, inviting written consent. The disabled person must be given ample time and opportunity to consider and discuss the request to ensure comprehension before giving an informed, written or witnessed verbal decision.

Non-therapeutic research

There are many health issues confronting young adults with physical disabilities which may prevent them from pursuing an active and independent life. At the same time research into these issues may be non-therapeutic – it may not be of direct, individual benefit, although it may be believed that it would serve to ameliorate situations for others with similar disabilities, perhaps in the future.

The ethical question of whether there should be an absolute prohibition against non-therapeutic research without consent is a controversial and difficult one. The Medical Research Council (MRC) recognises that,

> there are circumstances in which it is important to gain knowledge which may be of benefit to mentally incapacitated people in general and which can only be acquired as a result of research which involves those who are unable to consent.[12]

In such circumstances strong safeguards are necessary, and participants should be 'placed at no more than negligible risk of harm'.[13] The safeguards suggested by the MRC are as follows:

> those unable to consent should take part in research only if it relates to their condition and if the relevant knowledge could not be gained by research in persons able to consent

> all projects must be approved by the appropriate LREC(s) [local research ethics committees]

> the inclusion of an individual unable to consent should be subject to the agreement of an informed, independent person, acceptable to the LREC, that that individual's welfare and interests have been appropriately safeguarded

those included in the research do not object or appear to object in either words or action.[14]

However, the *legal* position may be somewhat at variance with what the MRC takes to be the ethical position. The individual, whether able-bodied or disabled, has certain legal rights. The MRC states that research 'must conform to all legal requirements' and, at the same time, that 'The legal position in relation to invasion of the human body and to consent to treatment and research is complex, and in many cases not clear.'[15]

The researcher may believe that consent of the relative or guardian will legally suffice. Indeed, the Declaration of Helsinki drawn up by the World Health Organisation in 1964 and most recently revised in 1983 states that: 'where physical or mental incapacity makes it impossible to give informed consent . . . permission from the responsible relative replaces that of the subject in accordance with National Legislation'.[16] However, national legislation in the UK is such that the consent of a relative, even that of the mother or father, is not recognised. The UK courts have not considered whether non-therapeutic research is under some conditions, however narrow, allowable in the public interest. The MRC takes quite a strong position on this issue:

> However, it seems to us that a case can be made out that it is not in the public interest for persons suffering from mental incapacity to be excluded from socially responsible behaviour purely through lack of consent competence. Where the risk attending participation in non-therapeutic research into mental disorder is minimal and a reasonable person with that disorder but able to consent is likely to accept that risk when told that such research might lead to advances in treatment, it would be strange if a person unable to consent because of that disorder should be imputed with a wholly different attitude to the welfare of the class of persons of which he is a member.[17]

This is a highly controversial area. It is quite understandable that many people would take the view that if a person cannot consent then no research of any kind should be permitted on that person. For my own part I think that nurses and nurse researchers working in this area, who generally have a closer familiarity with the capacities and problems of clients and their families, should be making a contribution to this debate. The issue is not a purely medical one. This is one area in which the ethics of nursing may prove to be rather different from, and equally as important as, the ethics of medicine.

Consent in our studies

The involvement of people with learning disabilities in our research investigation required careful consideration. The researcher had to take many interacting factors into account.

Before seeking participation, it was necessary to make some preliminary assessment of the individual client's cognitive function and ability to consent. Our sample of disabled people was recruited from charities and medical records and social service departments where information was usually recorded about their cognitive function and impairment. Some registers classify people with disabilities into the following: minor, moderate and severe learning difficulties. Some organisations advised us against writing to individuals with severe learning difficulties. Some charities proposed writing a preliminary letter on our behalf to those adults with minor to moderate learning difficulties known to them.

Our research team placed high priority in ensuring that people invited to participate in our study *were able* to give informed consent. Before interviewing the young person the researcher obtained permission to access information from the patient/client records about recent psychological assessments, general health status and educational attainment. All of these may be considered valuable indicators of cognitive function. Where the client's records were used to access biographical details prior consent to obtain such information was obtained. The Royal College of Nursing recognises that there may be practical difficulties in implementing this approach, not least for those with learning difficulties.[18]

All 100 invited participants in our studies were sent explanatory letters about the research and offered a preliminary interview to discuss their involvement. Six adults with disabilities requested a preliminary face-to-face interview and ten wanted an introductory telephone discussion prior to giving consent. Ten parents/carers requested preliminary discussions about the research on their son's or daughter's behalf. Four parents/carers refused consent on behalf of the young adult. Some parents opened their daughter's or son's mail and refused consent, sometimes without the young adult's knowledge. Two young adults requested that their parents be present at the interviews whilst three parents/carers asked to be present. Participants were offered the choice of a personal interview or to self-administer a questionnaire. The majority preferred, and took part in, a face-to-face interview.

There were considerable variations in the circumstances surrounding the disabled person's freedom to give consent. Some young people had total independence, others shared decision making with carers. Others never had the opportunity to know about the study, let alone discuss their feelings about it with the researcher. Cognition was not always the reason for denying the disabled person access to his/her correspondence. Many carers felt the subject matter was so sensitive that they preferred to 'protect' the disabled person from any 'undue stress' which might be prompted by the research.

CONFIDENTIALITY

Disclosure and responsibility

Clause ten of the UKCC's Code states that nurses, midwives and health visitors must,

> protect all confidential information concerning patients and clients obtained in the course of professional practice and make disclosures only with consent, where required by the order of a court or where you can justify disclosure in the wider public interest.[19]

There is often a great deal of misunderstanding about what is to be regarded as confidential information, and it may cause anxiety to health care professionals and even to lawyers. The object of confidentiality is:

> i) To respect the wishes of the person who imparted the confidence to you in that it was entrusted to you to facilitate care and treatment and for no other purpose.
> ii) In the wider interests of the profession, to ensure that patients/clients will continue to impart sensitive and confidential information to medical practitioners (where considered necessary).[20]

In practice there may be difficulties for the research nurse. The nurse seeks information, with consent, from the client for a research project – in this case from a disabled person participating in a sexuality study. The disabled person may impart sensitive and personal information to the researcher during the course of the interview. Some of the information may not be relevant to the research exercise but may be of considerable importance in safeguarding the client's future best interests. Several people in the sexuality study retrospectively disclosed rape, sexual abuse and the like. As the researcher I had to consider whether my clients were at further risk of abuse and consider my own responsibilities in the light of these disclosures, examining each case individually. Did I owe the client 'a duty of care' to impart this information to another agency to protect and safeguard the client's future interests, particularly if, for instance, the individual is immobile and unable physically to prevent further abuse? Or do I disclaim such responsibility on grounds such as the following: I would not have known of the abuse at all were it not for the research; the disclosures are mainly retrospective and the client is probably no longer at risk; imparting information to another agency at this stage may only initiate either inappropriate or unnecessary action and serve only to create further anxiety to the disabled person.

There may not be a simple answer. Researchers must consider their responsibilities in the light of the circumstances of each individual case. It is wrong to apply rules or guidelines for everyone in a blanket manner, particularly perhaps for disabled people. However, if I consider the client to be at risk of further abuse then I should obtain his or her consent to impart this information to an agency which may offer protection from further violation.

Access

Access to information about patients and clients is a sensitive subject. One may begin by asking, for whom is the research intended? The research subjects, the funding body, the researcher, or the employing body?

The funding body: in this case a charity which may wish to use the information to develop or review current service provision and the potential for expanding services.

The researcher: in pursuit of professional development, seeking an ethical research project to gain a postgraduate qualification.

The employing body: in my case a medical school, which may be as interested in auditing and developing research publications output as service provision for patients/ clients.

The research subjects: who not only provide the evidence on which to prove or refute the researcher's original hypotheses, but provide the rationale for doing the research in the first place. In an ethically informed science the information obtained belongs by right to all and should be accessible to all. Unfortunately, it happens too frequently that the people who provide the research data are the last to have access to it, to read it and to benefit from it.

The information should be disseminated in a style and form appropriate to the client, as well as in versions for other researchers, the employing authority or the funding body. On completing the sexuality study our department organised a seminar to present the survey results to young adults with disabilities. A video and accompanying leaflets were produced and also shown, describing some of the findings and recommendations.

If the researcher intends to use the research data and conclusions for teaching or private study (including, for example, material such as photographs, videos and audio tapes) then this intention must be made explicit and permission obtained both from the clients and the funding body. I well recall sitting in a lecture theatre with many others listening to a researcher presenting findings and feeling acutely uncomfortable when slides were shown of a client I recognised. I wondered if that client knew that personal information was being discussed with a large audience, albeit anonymously.

Most academic institutions hope that the research results will be worthy of publication, even if the original hypotheses are refuted. Many academic centres require an annual audit of publications. The researcher should not, however, feel coerced to publish or report within a defined timescale if he or she feels that additional time is needed to better serve clients and research objectives. Researchers must conform with the requirements of the ethics committee, and any amendments made to the original proposal during the course of investigation must be notified in writing to the chairperson of that committee.

ETHICS COMMITTEES

Recent reports and circulars have recommended that all general practice, dental, hospital and academic research within an area be considered by the LREC. The principal role of such committees is that of 'a public watchdog'; to safeguard and protect the interests of the general public, particularly those who are vulnerable such as children under the age of consent, the elderly and those with learning difficulties or mental impairment.[21] They also ensure that research participants are fully informed of research objectives, can give informed consent and are allowed the right to withdraw from research studies at any stage without anxieties.

The sexuality study which I pursued necessitated the recruitment of over 100 young adults with spina bifida and an equivalent number of able-bodied volunteers. The interviews took place in two regions but required the approval of over twenty individual medical ethics committees, despite the low number of people participating from each district. Over a third of the committees requested my presence at a meeting to answer questions and defend the protocol. In some cases this meant travelling distances over 50 miles and waiting several hours before the meeting occurred. One committee was inquorate on the day and cancelled the meeting upon my arrival asking me to come back a few weeks later.

I noted that the committee recommendations were often at variance. The impact of hydrocephalus on cognition and chronological age performance was a regular concern.

Whilst I fully support vigilance in approving research and close scrutiny of protocols, particularly with regard to a vulnerable group such as people with disabilities and learning difficulties, I maintain it would be helpful to researchers if there were some degree of standardisation for multicentred projects where only a relatively small number of people are recruited.[22]

CONCLUSION

All research involving the participation of human beings must be carefully planned, designed and well executed, with the welfare of the participants constantly in mind. Researchers must ensure that all contributors, but particularly those with physical and learning impairments, understand the full implications and significance of their involvement so that their acquired or congenital disabilities may not be exacerbated by any additional physical and/or emotional distress caused by their participation. Alderson has described research as,

> collecting data from people. They help us, and if we help them in return that is a bonus, but it is not the purpose of the encounter. The ethical responsibility is to remember this imbalance, the one

sidedness of research and our obligations to the people helping us.[23]

If we forget this principle, then we risk abusing the people who provide the information and deceive ourselves if we consider research always to be of mutual benefit.

Previously, research was mainly the domain of doctors. Nurses were not always informed or aware of research objectives. Many nurses merely assumed the role of data collectors for doctors and medical researchers without necessarily questioning their actions or responsibilities. Recent changes in nurse education have increased the awareness, interest, participation and initiation of research projects by nurses; particularly in therapeutic, cathartic counselling and psycho-social research.

Hinged on the research outcome is the recognition of professionalism, the trust, understanding, mutual respect and integrity established between the client and nurse, a relationship which is based on equality and recognition of the client's worth and contribution, regardless of their ability or disability.

ACKNOWLEDGEMENTS

My thanks go to the following: all the young adults who participated in the research; the Association for Spina Bifida and Hydrocephalus, for funding our research studies and allowing us to use some of the material in this chapter; Dr Martin C. O. Bax (Senior Research Fellow), Dr Clifford Strehlow (Research Fellow), Ms Yvonne Hunt (Research Assistant), Community Paediatric Research, Department of Child Health, Westminster Hospital, London; Dr Priscilla Alderson, Social Science Research Unit, Institute of Education, University of London; Mr Alan Hannah, Brachers Solicitors, Maidstone, Kent.

NOTES

1 See Jirovec. M. M., 'Research with Cognitively Impaired Older Adults: Issues of Informed Consent', *Michigan Nurse*, 1989, vol 62, pp. 6–15.
2 Edser, P. and Ward, G., 'Sexuality, Sex and Spina Bifida', in Bannister, C. M. and Tew, B., *Current Concepts in Spina Bifida and Hydrocephalus*, London: McKeith Press and Blackwell Scientific, 1991.
3 See Blackburn, M. C. and Bax, M.C.O., 'Sex Education Provision for Young Adults with Spina Bifida and/or Hydrocephalus: An Evaluation of a Pilot Training Video', *European Journal of Paediatric Surgery*,

1992, vol. 2 (Supp. 1), pp. 39–40; Blackburn, M.C., Bax, M.C.O., Strehlow, C. and Hunt, Y., 'Sexual Knowledge and Experiences of Young Adults with Spina Bifida and Hydrocephalus', Research Report for the Association of Spina Bifida and Hydrocephalus, 1994 (in press).

4 For a recent overview see Bannister and Tew, op. cit.

5 See Bancroft, J., *Human Sexuality and its Problems*, London: Churchill Livingstone, 1989.

6 Education Act 1986, para. 46 (2), (19). The World Health Organisation's International Classification of Impairments, Disabilities and Handicap (1980) gives these definitions of 'disability' and 'handicap':

   In the context of health experience, a disability is any restriction or lack (resulting from impairment) of ability to peform an activity in the manner or within the range considered normal for a human being.

   In the context of health experience, a handicap is a disadvantage for a given individual, resulting from an impairment or a disability, that limits or prevents the fulfilment of a role that is normal (depending on age, sex, and social and cultural factors) for that individual.

7 Dorner, S., 'Sexual Interest and Activities in Adolescents with Spina Bifida', *Journal of Child Psychology and Psychiatry*, 1977, vol. 18, pp. 229–37.

8 Masters, W. H. and Johnson, V. E., *Human Sexual Response*, London: J. & A. Churchill, 1966.

9 United Kingdom Central Council for Nursing, Midwifery and Health Visiting, *Code of Professional Conduct*, London: UKCC, 3rd edn, June 1992.

10 Thorpe, L., 'Informed Decision-Making', *Nursing*, 1989, vol. 3 (42), pp. 16–19.

11; Gunn, M., 'The Law and Mental Handicap: Consent to Treatment', *Mental Handicap*, 1985, vol 13, pp. 70–2.

12 Medical Research Council, *The Ethical Conduct of Research on the Mentally Incapacitated*, London: MRC, 1991, sec. 6.3.1.

13 ibid., sec. 6.3.2.

14 ibid., sec. 6.1.3. It is important to read this pamphlet as a whole.

15 Medical Research Council, *Responsibility in Investigations on Human Participants and Materials and on Personal Information*, London: MRC, 1992, pp. 8, 14.

16 World Medical Association Declaration of Helsinki, 1989, para. 1, sec. 11, reproduced in Department of Health, op. cit. (note 20 below), Appendix C.

17 Medical Research Council, op. cit., sec. 7.3.4.

18 Royal College of Nursing, *Issues in Nursing and Health*, London: RCN, 1992; No. 2: 'Patient Records and Research – A Position Statement', No. 3: 'Research Trials Advice for Nurses and Nursing Students', No. 6: 'Responding to Rape and Sexual Assault – Guidance for Good Nursing Practice', No. 9: 'Guidelines on Commercial Sponsorship', No. 16: 'Access to Health Records – The Nurse's Responsibility'.

19 UKCC, op. cit., sec. 10.

20 Hannah, A. I., 'Child Protection. The Way Forward: Some Legal Aspects of the Subject of Child Abuse', Greenwich Health Authority paper, 1989, pp. 2–3.
21 Department of Health, *Local Research Ethics Committees*, Heywood, Lancs.: Department of Health, 1991; Neuberger, J., *Ethics and Health Care: The Role of Research Ethics Committees in the United Kingdom*, London: King's Fund Institute, 1992; Hunt, G., 'Local Research Ethics Committees and Nursing: A Critical Look', *British Journal of Nursing*, 1992, vol. 1 (7), pp. 349–51.
22 The problem of ethical scrutiny of multicentre research is currently being considered by the Royal College of Physicians of London (RCP). See RCP, *Guidelines on the Practice of Ethics Committees in Medical Research Involving Human Subjects*, London: RCP, 1990, secs 13.18–13.19.
23 Alderson, P., *Children's Consent to Surgery*, Milton Keynes: Open University Press, 1993, ch. 5.

Chapter 6

Ethical issues in HIV/AIDS epidemiology

A nurse's view

Ann Kennedy

Nurses working in the field of HIV/AIDS epidemiology are often best placed to understand the anxieties, values, life problems, rights and obligations of sufferers. Yet they have very little voice in this field. As a nurse who has worked in the area for several years I hope to draw the attention of other health care professionals, nursing students and the public to some of the concerns which have arisen from my experience.

Nurses working in the epidemiological process often find themselves in morally problematic situations. Although the employment of nursing personnel in the data collection, record keeping and other disease surveillance aspects of epidemiology is widespread, the value and quality of their work is unrecognised and unrewarded.

The dilemmas nurses face in this position when issues such as consent and confidentiality are not properly aired and discussed can be severe. To offer an anecdote: when one of my nursing colleagues tried to discuss with doctors the issue of patients consenting to their personal details being reported to the surveillance centre she was simply told, 'If you don't want to do it, we'll just have to get someone else to do it.' My colleague was surprised to hear this from doctors who are well known for caring for people with HIV/AIDS at a London teaching hospital.

Practice sisters in GP group practices who often do the actual disease notification are not the ones to receive the statutory payment. Senior HIV/AIDS discharge co-ordinators (nurses) and research nurses have been employed with part of their job defined in terms which are normally part of the doctor's role. Needless to say, they are paid less than doctors.

There is generally a lack of recognition and concern for the dilemmas nurses are faced with in this field. Although the ethical codes of both the medical and nursing professions are not at odds on these matters, the actual practice is. In fact, I think the nursing code in particular is quite advanced and very clear, but the conflicts and power struggles which still exist between medicine and nursing make it very difficult for nurses – advocates of the patients – to live by the letter and spirit of their code.

Not only does the individual nurse suffer in this situation, but any decent nurse is forced into defending the rights of the patient in opposition to the quality of the data collected. This is not an argument against nurses entering the field of epidemiology, but rather an argument for bringing the rights of the individual patient and the public aims of epidemiology and health policy together. Nurses are often in the best position to identify these problems and should be listened to.

A SCENARIO

The scenario which follows is drawn from my own experience. It is realistic and not untypical. (The name and personal details have been changed.)

A question of confidentiality

A young woman, Amanda, is pregnant. She attends the antenatal clinic, where a midwife takes her health history and runs a series of tests, such as blood, urine and blood pressure. She is counselled by the midwife on, among other things, the implications of human immuno-deficiency virus (HIV) and of being tested for it. Although the midwife has no reason to believe that Amanda has been exposed to HIV, she offers her an HIV test. Amanda declines, as there seems to be no need for one. She is also aware of the difficulties in obtaining a mortgage if she has this test.

The blood sample taken by the midwife is sent to a laboratory for analysis for haemoglobin content, rubella antibodies, and syphilis. At the same time a small amount of blood from this sample is placed in an unnamed test tube which is then sent to a central laboratory to be tested for HIV. The midwife is completely unaware that this has occurred so cannot inform Amanda.

The next time that Amanda visits the antenatal clinic the other blood results are returned to her and, as they are normal, she continues with her pregnancy uneventfully. Unknown to her the anonymous blood sample has been tested and found to be HIV antibody positive and this is recorded at the national surveillance centre, where data on HIV and acquired immuno-deficiency syndrome (AIDS) and other infectious diseases are collected. The information accompanying this sample includes Amanda's age range (i.e. between 35 and 40 years), her gender and the geographical origin of the sample. In this case the epidemiologist will not have information about the means by which HIV was contracted. The data will provide information about the trends of HIV among pregnant women who attend antenatal clinics in an area of the UK over a five-year period.

Amanda's pregnancy continues normally and she delivers a healthy baby. The baby has a heel prick blood test (Guthrie Test), which is routinely performed on newborns to detect phenylketonuria (PKU) and hypothyroidism. In this case it includes a test for HIV. The PKU and hypothyroidism tests are linked to the baby's identity and are done with Amanda's knowledge, but the HIV test is anonymous and is done without her consent or knowledge.

Antibodies to HIV are detected, but it cannot be known whether these are 'maternal' antibodies circulating in the baby's bloodstream temporarily, eventually to disappear, or whether the baby actually has HIV infection. In any case, although this HIV antibody positive result contributes to more epidemiological evidence accumulating about HIV, no benefit has accrued, or can accrue, either to the baby or the mother from the test at this stage.

Amanda was not informed about either of the HIV tests and was not given the chance to decline or give her consent. So appropriate social and health benefits cannot be made available to Amanda, as she has no knowledge yet of her baby's or her own HIV antibody status.

The months pass by and Amanda begins to feel unwell. She develops swollen glands and experiences night sweats. On consulting her general practitioner (GP) a blood test is taken and a tentative diagnosis of glandular fever is made. Weeks go by and she returns for her result – negative. She is still ill and after much consideration and discussion her GP offers her an HIV test. The time waiting for the result is fraught with anxiety and the GP is apprehensive too. The test is positive, and so is a test on the baby's blood.

I will not discuss the quality of care which Amanda and her baby receive from the GP and the primary health care team. In fact it is excellent. Amanda, devastated by the news, is conscientiously supported by the team.

Time passes, and soon the various opportunistic infections which Amanda develops puts her in the 'AIDS' category.[1] Her GP informs her of this, although it makes very little difference to the care he gives her as she is treated for every infection according to the current practice. However, Amanda is troubled by this new label.

Meanwhile, a national surveillance system is in operation, and doctors are encouraged to report AIDS cases to a central surveillance unit. This is a voluntary system which began in 1982, and Amanda's GP fills in the appropriate form and sends it to the surveillance centre. Amanda is not aware of this procedure and the GP does not inform her. He does not think twice about it, after all, he reports many illnesses such as cytomegalovirus and legionnaire's disease on a voluntary basis. That is, these are not notifiable diseases, so there is no statutory requirement on the GP to report.

On receiving the report at the surveillance centre the epidemiologist, who is involved in a research study into routes of transmission of HIV, becomes interested in knowing how Amanda contracted HIV. Her GP had mentioned on the form that she was not a drug user, had not received infected blood products, and that she had said she had not behaved in a 'high risk manner'. (As she had no current sexual partner the GP felt it prudent not to delve any further.)

Approached through her GP, Amanda gives permission for the interview. The epidemiologist explains to her the purpose of the study. Amanda is interested not only in the reason for the interview but in how the interviewer had come by the information about her and her AIDS status. She is perplexed to learn that her GP, who had respected confidentiality so far, had sent information about her to a central surveillance unit without informing her or asking her permission. She begins to wonder how many other people know of her illness and whether this information is going to benefit her care or indeed be beneficial to any other people living with HIV or AIDS. She feels rather let down by her GP, but agrees to continue with the interview.

The interview takes several hours and she is asked very intimate questions about her sexual behaviour and history. The interviewer tries to establish whether the contact was only sexual, or whether it was with someone who had behaved in a 'high risk manner' (such as a drug user), whether the person was from a country where the heterosexual spread of HIV is common, whether her partner had been bisexual, or whether she had had a sexual partner about whose sexual history she was ignorant.

A question of trust

After reliving her past relationships in her mind Amanda became very upset. The interview brought up disturbing feelings which she had not acknowledged and had tried to suppress. Although the epidemiologist eventually got the information he wanted, it left Amanda feeling extremely confused and angry. After pinpointing the sexual partner from whom Amanda was most likely to have contracted HIV she felt very hostile towards him but directed this hostility towards her GP and the interviewer.

As Amanda's trust in the GP had now broken down he began to act defensively, and Amanda decided to complain to the interviewer's employers. She complained about what she regarded as a breach of confidentiality by the GP, as he had not asked for her consent to pass on the report, and also about the upsetting interview. The Medical Defence Union supported the GP, but the interviewer found himself unsupported by his professional body because he had not received formal ethical approval for the interview. He had in fact gone ahead with the research on the instructions of his superior. The rationale he offered for the absence of approval was that other field studies on disease outbreaks, such as legionnaire's disease, do not generally require ethical approval and, in any case, it was ultimately the responsibility of his superior.

However, it now seemed that the interviewer had breached his own professional code of conduct, for he was in fact responsible for all the relevant actions carried out by him whether ordered by his superior or not. He was wrong in thinking that his superior would have to carry the can alone. The director of the surveillance centre then gave Amanda an apology for the distress caused her and went on to explain how important and useful the information gained from her would be for the epidemiology of AIDS.

The investigations into why the study went ahead without ethical approval threw up some interesting issues, such as misunderstandings about the various roles and responsibilities of employees at the surveillance centre. These were compounded by the health workers having codes of conduct and ethical standards which, although not differing fundamentally, led to different interpretations. Not only was the role of the ethical committee called into question, but its composition and representativeness and its understanding and application of the various codes were now being queried by some. There was some consideration of the reluctance with which members of the surveillance centre submitted studies for ethical scrutiny, and it was discovered that many feared rejection of their studies. This led either to their seeking ethical approval elsewhere or carrying out studies without ethical approval.

I will now consider five themes of moral concern which emerge from this scenario. The themes are:

1 The anonymous HIV antibody test done on Amanda's blood at the antenatal clinic without her consent.
2 The anonymous HIV antibody test done on Amanda's baby without consent.
3 The GP's report on Amanda's AIDS status to the national surveillance centre, without her consent and possibly breaching confidentiality.
4 The circumstances of the epidemiologist's interview.
5 The conduct of a research study (of which the interview was a part) without ethical approval.

CONSENT FOR AMANDA'S TEST

When a woman attends an antenatal clinic it is with the tacit understanding that she will be screened for various disorders which may affect the antenatal or future health of herself or her baby. She expects that in good faith she will be notified about any abnormalities which are detected during her visits, in order that she or her attendant midwives or doctors can take appropriate action. If this does not occur then she may rightly consider that there has been a breach of trust, a shortcoming in the duty of care.

In this case a pregnant woman attends the clinic with trust, but without the knowledge that in fact non-therapeutic research is being carried out on her blood sample. Surely there is an element of deception here, and this is made more complex if the staff in the clinic, including nurses and midwives, are also ignorant of the existence of an anonymous testing programme. As deception is generally wrong, one might ask whether there are instances when it is nevertheless justified. Certainly it is not immediately clear how this particular deception can harm patients or staff, but that may not be the crucial point.

It would appear that neither harms nor benefits can come to Amanda from the anonymous screening programme. When the epidemiologists have the data they cannot be directly linked in any way back to Amanda (or anyone in the same position as her) and therefore can neither harm nor benefit her. The programme will, it is assumed, benefit the epidemiologists, by giving them material to write about, publish articles, expand their CVs and enhance their career prospects. It may also increase the body of knowledge about HIV and AIDS, although it is a further question whether this is knowledge which will one day bring advantage to sufferers.

To consider the possible benefits which might be gained from the data which accrue from anonymous testing without consent, one must examine their quality and value. If there were grounds for foreclosing consent (for example, because it introduces bias into the data) and at the same time the data to be obtained would be very valuable, then it might be considered justifiable to go ahead without consent. Here one might think of consent, as important as it is, being overridden by the great value of the data and the importance of minimising bias. Presumably the value of the data would reside in their possible contribution to planning for the care of people with HIV and AIDS in future years. The argument, then, is that knowledge of the rate of change of prevalence of HIV in the community might justify the carrying out of a study without the consent of patients (or staff).

It might be decided that, should the change in prevalence of HIV in the community be below a certain threshold, then one plan for care and resources would be put into operation and, should the change be above a certain threshold, then a different plan would be implemented, and so on. However, as far as I have been able to ascertain, this is not the case and epidemiologists and others involved have no such plans. Therefore, relying on the argument about the value of the information is not at present a justification for collecting HIV prevalence data without consent. (Indeed, one may wonder whether it provides a justification for collecting the information at all, even with consent.)

The nurses involved should not be hoodwinked into thinking that epidemiologists and those they advise have some superior but unstated knowledge such that nurses should participate in foreclosing consent in dealing with their patients and clients.[2] Having said that, I accept that if there were data which would be valuable in relating to specific plans then it is just possible, under some circumstances, that proceeding with anonymous testing without consent might be justified. But a careful and openly debated case would have to be made for this.

In looking at why consent was not considered important in this particular study two reasons appear to have been paramount. First, in performing an HIV test on people who have been informed it is accepted in health care circles that they must receive counselling before and after the test. To avoid this and all the cost and education necessary the planners stated that in the government's view there would be no legal or ethical objections to anonymous screening without consent. It was said that if the blood samples were anonymous then there would be no reason to obtain consent. (As far as I can see, no legal sources have ever been quoted to support this.)

Second, it was assumed that if people were asked they would often refuse to give consent even to an anonymous test for HIV, and that this would bias the study. However, this was assumed without even a pilot study being carried out to determine what the refusal rate would be and whether it would introduce bias. I believe this might have provided a golden opportunity for public education and a great chance to be effective in changing attitudes and behaviour and thereby helping to prevent the spread of HIV.

One might have expected that at least the health care personnel involved would be fully informed. However, in practice this would amount to informing the patients, because the nurses and midwives would have had a professional duty to inform their patients and clients. This would have led to a demand for consent procedures. Alternatively, nurses and midwives might have been pressured to ignore this duty, which would have been unethical and created enormous difficulties. It seems to me that the foreclosing of consent, and the withholding of information, both from patients or clients and from health care staff, shows a lack of respect for both groups.

As a nurse working in epidemiology, yet independent of its interests, it is clear to me that the very idea that pregnant women represent the 'heterosexual population' is misconceived. I propose the alternative of anonymous screening with consent, which would also have the epidemiological advantage of allowing matching of data with the current demographic data from an area. This way the patient/client is respected, the chance to give or refuse consent is allowed and, should people refuse, some sensitive non-threatening enquiries could follow into the reasons for refusal, reasons which may themselves be enlightening for educational purposes. My view of the wrongness of the screening programme resides in my role as a nurse, a role which demands of me, through my professional code of conduct, that I exercise accountability, guided by considerations of truth and consent, and act always as the advocate of patients and clients.[3]

CONSENT FOR THE BABY'S TEST

Amanda was not asked whether or not she would like her baby to be tested for HIV. The baby's blood was tested anonymously, so although the epidemiologists know that somewhere there is a baby with HIV antibodies they do not know who that baby is so cannot offer information or help. Amanda's baby may not be personally tested or diagnosed for some time after the Guthrie test and may miss out on essential preventive measures, or treatment and care which may prolong life or make it more comfortable.

Here the question of a duty of care might arise. Is there not a failure of duty in not offering the baby, through her mother, a service which might crucially affect the baby's life? Simply asking the mother this question may have aroused feelings which would have led her to reconsider a test for herself at that stage. But she was denied this opportunity.

What Priscilla Alderson has to say is relevant here:

> Moral feeling such as compassion is essential to informed proxy consent, given by parents on behalf of their child. Compassion arouses anxiety which may be dismissed as an emotion that prevents people thinking clearly. Yet only through enduring anxiety and thinking out what it means, can we appreciate the real significance of the risk which we consent to undertake.[4]

CONFIDENTIALITY AND THE GP'S REPORT

Practice nurses should be familiar with the AIDS surveillance form filled in by GPs. In the scenario the GP had a choice of putting down Amanda's name or using a code, and he chose a code. This is an alpha numeric code, which cannot be decoded easily, and thus provides a degree of confidentiality. However, the GP also fills in the form with Amanda's date of birth, address, occupation, sexual preference, route of transmission of HIV, if known, and various clinical details such as when she became HIV antibody or antigen positive, when she developed AIDS and what infections she has which fulfil the case definition of AIDS.

I do not say that submitting this information is prima facie wrong, but I do think that submitting it without her knowledge and consent is wrong.

It might be asked, however, whether this is a case of sharing privileged information within the bounds of a profession, which would appear to be an acceptable practice. But this practice is itself justified in terms of improving the care of the patient. I maintain that at the present stage in the history of this illness (HIV/AIDS is about ten years old), it cannot be regarded as being like other diseases and should not be treated as such from the point of view of surveillance and confidentiality. However much one would like to see the disappearance of the discrimination and stigma surrounding it, the present reality is far from that. Given that reality, confidentiality is of very great concern to people with HIV infection and AIDS. It is an issue which has been taken very seriously by the United Kingdom Central Council for Nursing, Midwifery and Health Visiting (UKCC) in a special document which spells out the necessity for gaining consent from patients before information is disclosed. The exceptions are: 'when the disclosure is required by law or by the order of a court or is necessary in the public interest'.[5]

Although confidentiality is stressed in medical ethics the legal protection available for health information not related to AIDS is limited – unlike some European countries, the disclosure of confidential medical information is not a crime in the UK. In civil law there is a duty of confidentiality, and a patient could claim damages for economic loss resulting from breach of confidence. However, when the Law Commission looked at the issue in 1981, they thought it unlikely that claims for mental distress resulting from disclosure of medical information would succeed. The Commission did recommend that a breach of 'such usual confidences as arise between doctor and patient' should be an offence, but this has not been adopted.

The National Health Service (Venereal Diseases) Regulations 1974 impose a specific duty of confidentiality on health authorities as far as sexually transmitted diseases are concerned. AIDS and HIV would be covered, but have not been tested in law. Under the regulations, health authorities must take all necessary steps to prevent disclosure of the identity of people examined or treated for sexually transmitted diseases unless disclosure is to a doctor or someone employed under a doctor's direction and is for the purpose of treating or preventing a disease. They relate only to health authorities and not to NHS general practitioners or private practices.

It is here that I wish to highlight the confusion between, on the one hand, privileged information-sharing in a sexually transmittable diseases clinic in order that the patient is properly and holistically cared for and, on the other, the practice of reporting cases of AIDS to an epidemiological centre for surveillance purposes. Since the HIV/AIDS reporting practice does not relate to prevention, treatment or care for an individual there is no ethical basis for the non-consenting and privileged information-sharing practice. Certainly such a practice is of great moral concern to nurses and some doctors involved in HIV/AIDS work.

There is a recent example of a public breach of confidentiality in which the legal judgement firmly established the right to confidentiality of people with AIDS. This is the case of x versus y (1987), in which the court granted a permanent injunction to stop a tabloid newspaper from publishing the names of two doctors with AIDS. What the judge said is interesting. He decided that confidentiality is of paramount importance for people with AIDS, and that if confidentiality is breached people would be reluctant to come forward for counselling and treatment. If this happened then the public would suffer through the increasingly rapid spread of the infection. Thus the public interest in preserving confidentiality for people with AIDS was held to outweigh substantially the public interest in the freedom of the press to publish such information. This ruling strengthened the law on confidentiality since publishing the names of people with the disease without their permission could now be an act of contempt of court and thus a breach of criminal law as well as of civil responsibility.[6]

What has been decided legally is that HIV/AIDS is to be treated with great sensitivity and not like a notifiable disease (because notification would discourage risk groups from seeking advice), and yet in practice the disease is being treated like a notifiable disease precisely because patients are not informed or consulted about personal information.

It may well be that people with HIV/AIDS have a moral duty to make this known to appropriate bodies. After all, it is within the ability, and part of the responsibility, of an individual to help prevent the transmission of the disease to others. But surveillance can do nothing to encourage this unless infected people are informed of the reporting activities and given a chance to understand the benefits of the system while also understanding the dangers. They could then discuss with the reporter the sensitivity of the information and the amount and kind of information which they feel prepared to pass on. As a nurse, working directly with patients and therefore aware of their personal situation, and fears and hopes, it seems obvious to me that here is an opportunity for education, co-operation and the building of trust.

How different things might have been for Amanda if she had had the chance to discuss with her GP the possibility of reporting.

THE INTERVIEW

Does the need to obtain information on how Amanda contracted HIV justify the deep upset which it caused her? If the information gathered were valuable in the way I discussed earlier then perhaps it is justified, but I threw doubt on this value. Did Amanda give informed consent to the interview; did she really grasp what it would involve? Would the interview procedure and the upsetting of the interviewee have been justified if the study had received ethical approval? Does it matter that the relationship between Amanda and her GP may have been jeopardised by the surveillance process and the interview? Do the interviews create more problems than they solve?

It is not clear what the root cause of the upset was. Possibly it was the knowledge that Amanda's GP had sent the information to the surveillance centre without her knowledge, or perhaps the way in which the interview forced her to focus on the person who probably passed the virus to her. Perhaps it was a combination of factors. What is clear is that she felt that she was not herself the primary concern in the whole matter.

The aim of the interview was purely epidemiological. She should already have been counselled by a health visitor or counsellor, and they should have discussed the possible source of her HIV and how she should protect future partners by using safe sex practices. Attempts should also have been made by this time for appropriate support personnel or contact with self-help groups. These would not be aims of the interviewer. In fact, he may not have shown any concern for these at all.

Let us return to the question of the value of the interview. Several arguments could be presented for its usefulness and I touched on some of these earlier. However, without going too deeply into these here, I maintain that its value is questionable because the aim is misguided. The epidemiological approach attempts to categorise people according to the membership of some 'high risk group', or more exactly in terms of risky behaviour. This strategy seems to me to indicate an ignorance of actual sexual behaviour, and possibly 'homophobia' and a political decision made in the early days of the epidemic to group, for example, gay and bisexual men in the same category.

It soon became apparent to some in the field that those belonging to, or identifying with, the gay scene were taking drastic steps to change their social and sexual behaviour to prevent HIV transmission. Some time later it became obvious with more education and understanding of human sexual behaviour, that homosexual and bisexual behaviour are not of the same type. Yet no move has been made to separate these risk behaviour categories so that changes can be studied. Some men who live in heterosexual relationships and see themselves as heterosexual can behave in a homosexual way. That is, they have a bisexual life-style but their sexual identity is heterosexual. If the observation of a heterosexual increase in the epidemic is being masked by including bisexual men in the gay category then this could be very misleading.

I would ask if what we have here is a lack of understanding of the existence of a continuum in human sexuality ranging from homosexual to heterosexual, so that some people are definitely one or the other all their lives while others fall somewhere in between for various periods? Or is it a politically motivated oversight, which has the aim of reducing the apparent heterosexual spread of HIV?

Consistency and clarity in research design and data analysis are important if the data are to be truly representative. If the information gathering exercise, such as interviewing, is to be worthwhile then an effort must be made flexibly to reclassify and group separately the sexual behaviours. Without a preparedness to rethink the epidemiological strategy, people like Amanda may be made upset and anxious without good reason. In actuality it seems that Amanda was merely used as a means to a poorly conceived end.

The threat to the good relationship Amanda had with her GP could have been prevented. Had he informed her of the report, then she may have been more favourably disposed to the interviewer. He too may have approached her with greater respect.

I will also mention here the personal difficulties which arise for health care professionals themselves. After all, they have a duty, not just to collect information, but to care for the people they are gathering information from. Certainly, collecting information, especially by interview, in these special circumstances, cannot be done by people who have no caring role whatsoever – like census interviewers – who can remain completely detached. A training in bereavement counselling and listening skills is of great value but does not adequately answer the question of how to care for the carer. Unfortunately this is a problem many employers do not wish to hear about. Nurses in particular are often under great strain. I would suggest that perhaps the employer has a moral responsibility to provide adequate support to research workers who are involved in highly emotive, and grief-laden situations.

On balance I think the interview process in the present context, with all its ramifications, creates more problems than it resolves. Although the upset and anxiety may not have been completely prevented, still the conduct of the interview could have been quite different if Amanda had consented to the GP's report instead of just being automatically recorded as an 'AIDS case', and if the research protocol had been properly examined by an ethical committee. I now turn to the latter.

ETHICAL APPROVAL

Submission of the research study to an ethical committee at the Public Health Laboratory Service may not have entirely obviated the causing of upset to Amanda, but it may have minimised it. This would depend on how good that committee was. An ethics committee, if it approved the interview research at all, might have demanded that it be made sensitive enough to have ensured that the interviewer was better prepared for his delicate task.

The absence of official ethical approval for the research study is a prima-facie wrong. I will consider here the question of whether epidemiological surveillance can properly be regarded as research, and whether HIV and AIDS can be considered to have the same moral and ethical connotations as other diseases, notifiable or not. I will also touch on the ethical problems which are highlighted by a research nurse working in epidemiology, such as myself, and governed by a strict code of conduct, who has to work with doctors and others who may simply not see the moral aspects.

It might be argued that surveillance is not research, that this is generally undertaken without official ethical approval and that in any case epidemics require rapid responses which the approval process would obstruct.

First, I would question the assumption that the surveillance of disease in general does not require ethical approval. I think we should assume that surveillance of any disease, notifiable or not, requires such approval unless some overriding reason can be provided. If urgency does not permit a scrutiny of each and every study, then perhaps a standard approach could be agreed in which policy decisions are made public. For example, the policy that consent will be obtained, or will not be obtained in such and such circumstances for such and such reasons, or that people will always be informed of surveillance activities, or that confidentiality will be respected by such and such means.

Second, even if HIV/AIDS does come to be regarded as 'ordinary' as any other disease under surveillance, it is still true that at present it remains very much an 'unknown' and stigmatised disease surrounded by taboo. People living with HIV/AIDS suffer degrees of discrimination not experienced by the sick since the time of bubonic plague and leprosy. People with HIV/AIDS have to be protected, since they can be greatly damaged by the unbridled discrimination which is prevalent in all parts of the world. In these early years of this pandemic, health carers should be aware of these problems and strive to minimise the harm which can be caused by ignorance and insensitivity; and properly constituted ethical committees can go a long way in achieving this.

There still appears to be little control over and standardisation of ethical review committees in the UK. Membership is often arbitrary and standards of review vary from one health authority to another. Where in one committee one might get a study refused in another one might get approval with perfunctory 'chairman's approval'. Hopefully the recent Department of Health guidelines on ethical review committees will improve the situation.[7]

However, I feel it is time for a national statutory body to review health related research in the UK, on which there is active nursing representation. Countries such as Australia have a Federal Government Medical Research Ethics Committee and a Federal AIDS

Research Review Committee, but the British government recently reconfirmed its view that 'medical ethics' is a matter for the profession and not for government. In parliament Mrs A. Clwyd asked for 'a statement on medical ethics in practice and protection for patients against unscrupulous operations'. The response was:

> It is for the medical profession itself, and in particular the General Medical Council to lay down ethical guidance for doctors taking into account the changing attitudes in society, and to ensure that it is followed. Such guidance applies equally to private practice as for practice in the NHS.[8]

I do not think this is good enough. I share with others the view that the UK should adopt a system similar to that which is in place in the United States.[9] Levine says:

> Although the goals of ethical review in the US and Britain are identical, there are some striking contrasts in the means employed to pursue them. In the US, but not in Britain, ethical review and approval is required by national law for most types of clinical research; virtually all research institutions have negotiated agreements with the federal government that extend the requirement for ethical review to all clinical research.[10]

US federal regulations specify minimum requirements for membership, functions and operations of the institutional review board (the American name for an ethical committee). The ethical criteria for approval of research by these boards are set forth in considerable detail in federal regulations. The boards have the authority to monitor the conduct of research to ensure compliance with standards. If they detect non-compliance or 'unexpected serious harm to subjects' they are empowered to suspend or terminate the research.

Nursing and ethical review

I would like to ask: to whom are the British ethical committees presently accountable, and how are their important responsibilities exercised, monitored and controlled? I doubt that there are satisfactory answers at present. I would hope that nurses in particular will come to apply pressure for the reform of ethical review in the UK. After all, as advocates of patients and clients they may have a special responsibility in this regard.

There is another issue which nurses need to raise here. Many of the matters raised in this chapter could be the subject of further research by nurses, acting on the basis of patient advocacy. But very often ethical committees are dominated by medical personnel, and even if there is a nursing representative on the committee it may be unable to deal adequately with nursing research. Nurses have a different training, a professional code of their own, judgements and aims of their own and often a special concern for and identification with patients, clients and subjects.

I appreciate that the epidemiological surveillance of HIV/AIDS for the purpose of public health is a team effort, a team comprising epidemiologists, medical doctors, non-medical doctors, scientists, statisticians, nurses, midwives, health visitors and others. But what continues to be an underlying concern for many nurses such as myself is the apparent lack of regard for the ethical issues involved.

My own personal experience in this field has been that when I expressed ethical concerns about an HIV/AIDS project the research was delayed because the appropriate submission to the ethical committee was unnecessarily delayed. That I, as the only nurse, should have been the sole person concerned about the ethical issues arising in a medically run organisation is very worrying. I was disappointed that after pursuing my concerns as far as I could through the appropriate ethical committee I still had to turn to the UKCC where only informal ethical comments were offered. This was an unenviable path to have to follow, casting me in the unwilling role of 'troublemaker' and threat to the establishment.

There is something very wrong if nursing values and medical and epidemiological research come into conflict in this way.

The St Thomas' Hospital research

While I was reworking this chapter a piece of research was published of a character which realises some of the fears I have been expressing. In 1992, four years after the initial anonymous screening of pregnant women began in the UK, a letter was published in *The Lancet* on the HIV sero-prevalence among pregnant women.[11] The authors claim that by using unlinked anonymous testing they found a nine-fold increase in the prevalence of HIV infection among women attending antenatal clinics at St Thomas' Hospital, London between 1988 and 1990. They state, 'Among these patients there was a high proportion of women classified in their notes as being from ethnic minority groups, including women originating from west or central Africa.'

The authors are interested in identifying risk factors so that HIV/ AIDS health care resources can be 'targeted accurately'. They state that they obtained local ethics committee approval to look again at the serum obtained from women attending antenatal clinics in 1990, this time linking the serum to ethnic origin, age and history of injecting drug use of patient and partner. Having taken this step they then assumed that the presence of malarial antibodies and hepatitis B virus core antibodies in the serum is a marker of 'either recent travel to, or of having been raised in, endemic areas'. Because the authors found that malarial antibodies were detected in nine of ten HIV positive patients in the 'African ethnic origin' group they conclude that this suggests 'these patients may have acquired their HIV infection in Africa rather than in the UK'.

The authors conclude that 'consideration be given to initiating testing on a named basis' in antenatal clinics. But since it would be 'invidious to target HIV testing at specific ethnic categories', as well as inefficient, universal testing should be introduced.

In the light of what I have already said in previous sections, this study is quite worrying. Did the ethics committee make the right decision? Did the patients give consent to having their blood tested? Did they consent to having it re-examined? Would the patients have given consent if they had known the samples would be identified to the whole world by ethnic origin, age and history of injecting drug use? Did the members of these groups subsequently become anxious, and will this anxiety lead them to volunteer for tests, tests which in the present climate may damage their prospects?

The researchers maintained anonymity and 'ensured the impossibility of deductive disclosure of HIV positivity by removing all identifying data (name and hospital number) from serum before testing, and maintaining subgroup sizes of more than 20'. But does mere anonymity guarantee confidentiality when so much circumstantial information is disclosed? The individuals may not have been named, but the groups to which they belong have, in a sense, been named.

The women and children involved may live in the UK and need to be cared for there. Even if the assumptions are valid, and the scientific design is acceptable (which I doubt), what use is the knowledge of the country of contraction of HIV when the care of those infected is likely to be in the UK? The health education for prevention of further transmission from these women cannot begin if they are not aware of their HIV sero-status. What harm may the publication, and the surrounding media publicity, have caused in increasing prejudices against ethnic minorities?

The nurses and midwives involved in the research are left in a difficult position. The St Thomas' Hospital medical researchers may be criticised for not gaining proper approval from all the staff.

Two of the researchers, Banatvala and Smith, later accepted that 'a small group of women has been made uncomfortable', but Smith is quoted as saying that 'this was not a matter for the ethics committee'.[12]

CONCLUSION

It should be possible to learn from mistakes made in the historical past during great epidemics and resist public health measures which are crude and unthinking. The deception and secrecy and breaches of human rights which tend to occur in these situations, either intentionally or unintentionally, cannot be justified even in the case of HIV/AIDS. With changes in attitudes and ethical awareness epidemiologists could produce surveillance and research programmes which respect consent, confidentiality and other rights. This would not make the control of the epidemic more difficult, it would make it easier.

The focus should be taken off the need to test and quantify HIV/ AIDS sero-positive individuals. Harvey Fineberg, Dean of the Harvard School of Public Health, stated recently that the 'emphasis is moving from testing for public health efforts in preventing spread, to tests being used for the benefit of the patient'.[13]

At the moment the only means of preventing or reducing the spread of HIV which has any success lies at the level of the individual. The course of the epidemic will be determined by what changes each individual is prepared to make to his or her sexual behaviour. Therefore the public health authorities cannot afford to alienate individuals with high-handed and insensitive behaviour on their part. Nurses, I believe, have a vital role to play in bringing public health policies and administration closer to the people.

NOTES

1 Centres for Disease Control, 'Revision of the CDC Surveillance Case Definition of Acquired Immuno-Deficiency Syndrome', *Morbidity and Mortality Weekly Report*, 1987, vol. 36, Supplement no. 1S.

2 This article is based on my unpublished MA dissertation, 'In the Name of Epidemiology: The Surveillance of HIV and AIDS', 1989, University of Wales. Further elaboration of and support for my arguments can be found here. In particular my criticisms of the protocol for the surveillance 'route of transmission' project are to be found on pp. 19 ff.

3 See the following UKCC documents: *Code of Professional Conduct* (1992); *Exercising Accountability* (1989) and *Confidentiality* (1987); Annexa (RHP/CS 2) to Registrar's Letter 8/1992, a Council Position Statement on AIDS and HIV Infection (1992).

4 Alderson, P., 'Trust in Informed Consent', *IME Bulletin* (Institute of Medical Ethics), 1988, no. 40, pp. 17–19.

5 See UKCC, *Confidentiality*, op. cit., and Institute of Medical Ethics, 'Medical Confidentiality', *Briefings in Medical Ethics*, 1990, no. 7, pp. 1–4.

6 X v Y, in *The Times*, 7 November 1987. See also Lee, S., 'Judges, Human Rights and the Sources of Medical Law', in P. Byrne (ed.), *Health, Rights and Resources: King's College Studies 1987–88*, London: King Edward's Hospital Fund for London, 1988, pp. 53–4.

7 Department of Health, *Local Research Ethics Committees*, Heywood, Lancs.: Department of Health, 1991 (HSG(91)5).

8 Hansard 240489, col. 327.

9 See Warnock, M., 'A National Ethics Committee', *British Medical Journal*, 1988, vol. 297, pp. 1626–7.

10 Levine, R.J., *The Ethics and Regulation of Clinical Research*, Baltimore, USA: Urban & Schwarzenberg, 2nd edn, 1986.

11 Chrystie, I. L., Palmer, S. J., Kenney, A. and Banatvala, J. E., 'HIV Sero-prevalence among Women Attending Antenatal Clinics in London', *The Lancet*, vol. 33 (8 February 1992), p. 364.

12 See De Selincourt K., 'A Breach of Trust?', *Nursing Times*, 1992, vol. 88 (11), p. 19.

13 Fineberg, H., 'Screening and Public Health Policy', The Second International Conference on Health Law and Ethics, plenary session paper, 1 July 1989, London.

Part II

General issues

Chapter 7

Nursing accountability

The broken circle

Geoffrey Hunt

The most fundamental question for anyone considering ethical practice in nursing is whether such a thing is possible. Particular ethical concerns arise where there is responsibility, and responsibility presupposes freedom. It is still far from clear whether nurses in the UK are free to judge and act as carers – and scrutiny of this leads one to fall back on the deeper question of what a nurse *is*. Even in the USA and Canada, where nursing is said to be 'more independent' of medicine, the root question is still how far it is actually independent and in what ways?

Even to raise the question of nursing's independence is still quite novel, certainly unorthodox and perhaps revolutionary. The subordinate nature of nursing was established in the last century. As Jane Salvage succinctly put it: 'The growth of "scientific medicine" and its development in hospitals created a need for doctors to have assistants who would do their bidding and keep the place in order.' While nursing gained in stature as it took on a clearer identity with the reforms of Florence Nightingale, the question of its independence was hardly touched. 'Florence Nightingale's belief that patients needed nursing care, spiritual support and a healthy environment was subsidiary to the doctors' requirements.'[1] The Nurses, Midwives and Health Visitors Act 1979 was regarded by some as the herald of a new era of professional nursing, a kind of 'liberation'. Reginald Pyne of the new nurses' regulatory body, the United Kingdom Central Council for Nurses, Midwives and Health Visitors (UKCC) said, 'There can be no doubt that this is legislation that is not about going backwards or simply standing still. It is most certainly about going forward.'[2] But in what way has nursing gone forward in the fifteen years since the Act?

If nursing is a 'mediated profession', the executive arm of a 'true' profession (medicine) then accountability cannot be expected of it except in what might be called the *military* sense. To be accountable in this sense is scrupulously to follow orders, as a soldier does.[3]

The subordinate role of nursing is also unquestionably tied up with the subordinate role of women generally, for it is still true that the overwhelming majority of nurses are women while the overwhelming majority of those who give them instructions (doctors, managers) are men. Thus the basic ethical question of nursing – its moral freedom – is also the ethical question of gender.[4]

ACCOUNTABILITY – AN IDEOLOGY?

The talk of accountability in nursing which began with the 1979 Act has intensified of late.[5] Managers, particularly nurse managers, speak of it frequently, nurse educators give classes with this theme and professional bodies re-emphasise its importance. The average nurse still appears to believe that accountability is all about *following procedure* and making sure that 'one is covered' by having the right kind of note or record or witness to refer to when something goes wrong or when, for whatever reason, an accusation is made. Still, one does hear from many that there is more to it than this – but what? What does 'accountability' mean? What is at the bottom of all this talk? This is the question which I shall address here, in very general terms.

Talk of accountability arises with the fundamental transformation which nursing is undergoing in the UK and some other European countries. The transformation that it is actually undergoing may not be the same that is officially claimed. In fact, it is still too early to say definitely what kind of transformation this is, except that it already appears that the age-old gap between nursing ideals and practice is taking yet another form. On the one hand, it would appear that 'accountability' is about the liberation of nurses, about a new freedom, responsibility and professionalism. On the other, the evidence is of 'accountability' functioning as the central idea in a new ideology of disciplined accommodation to structural changes required by a quasi-market in public health care provision. The year of the new Act was also the year that *laissez-faire* ideology was resurrected and put on the offical agenda by a New Right government in the UK.

There is a deep ambivalence in the use of the term. Put a cross-section of the health care hierarchy around a table and very often you will find them disagreeing about almost everything, only finally to agree about the importance of accountability. It appears that here is a concept serving an ideological function, one which papers over deep conflicts of interest. In a reversal of the story about blindfolded people feeling an elephant, all of whom come up with different ideas about the object before them, here everyone thinks they have an elephant when they are really feeling quite different animals.

Demanding 'accountability' does not in itself say anything about whom one is accountable to, or who has the right to hold one to account. It neither says what things one is, or ought to be, account-able for, nor what the limit to these things is. It does not say by what criteria, or on what basis, one is held to account. There will be many contexts in which demands for accountability come into conflict with one another. And it is often important to distinguish between the accountability of an individual and that of a group or institution.

One suspects that the recent talk of accountability is for the most part an absorption of nursing into a more thoroughly technical-rational understanding of health and health care.[6] Hence the in-creasing employment of administrative techniques and instruments such as QALYs (Quality Adjusted Life-Years), Audit, Quality Assurance and other measuring devices in understanding needs, delivery and distribution. Accountability is here tied up with the increasing technicalisation of care.[7]

The existing political and ideological *background* to health care accountability pre-empts the very question which is most in need of an answer: what is the moral basis of nursing? If nursing is about executing the orders of the biomedical (and increasingly the eco-nomic) expert then it follows that a whole series of fundamental ethical questions have been pre-empted. It appears, for instance, that there are two kinds of people, experts and lay, and to be accountable to the lay is necessarily secondary to being accountable to one's professional and managerial superiors. Thus while the health care professional may feel some obligation to give an explan-ation to a patient, if the patient does not accept it then the presumption is that the patient is *ignorant*. Patients, far from determining the character of health care are, for the most part, merely tolerated.

Although the word 'obedience' is generally avoided with some embarrassment one has to ask whether it is still in actuality the first principle of nursing practice, as was openly avowed at the turn of the century.[8] Despite the progress achieved by the nursing process, and the challenge of holistic nursing, there seems ever to be a tendency for nursing to slip back into a practice exhaustively definable in a set of *procedures*. But what causes this perennial tendency? The whole character and meaning of this set of procedures is determined from outside nursing itself by forces and agencies which nursing has never been prepared to consider or confront.

Nursing theorists have on the whole created conceptual frameworks for nursing in a political, economic and ethical vacuum and this inevitably stamps their theories with artificiality and consigns them to irrelevance. Nursing cannot be rethought and reshaped *independently* of a recognition and understanding of the realities of its position *vis-à-vis* medicine, economic management and political bureaucracy.

Doctors, of course, do have a conceptual framework (predominantly outdated positivistic science) and by means of this, or through it, they are able to define and interpret 'findings' (normality, risk, diagnosis and prognosis). In this framework the doctors appear as the 'experts' who, being just that, do not need to justify themselves further – accountability is apparently not really their problem (putting aside issues of malpractice, such as having sex with a patient).[9]

This however accounts for the patients' experience of professionals as people who 'know a lot' of arcane matters but ignore (or even deny) other things which they know as ordinary people (fathers, brothers, friends, lovers, husbands, citizens, etc.) and which are of even greater importance but do not fit into the framework. As the mother of a handicapped child says:

> I just think that ordinary people find it easier to accept the [Down's Syndrome] children for what they are, and expect things from them, and to change their attitudes if they had any previous [negative] attitudes. Whereas professional people don't seem to be able to accept them as human beings: they seem to be a case number, you know, 'mentally handicapped', not much going for them. They [professionals] seem to be immovable, whereas friends and people in the public that you meet, you can talk to them.[10]

Nurses have always been put under the constant pressure of trying to understand their work in terms of this same framework, although it can make little sense of it. One cannot *care* for people as the mere instrument of the biomedical (or economic) expert. In the light of this subordinate role one can see why 'accountability' is presented as a problem for nursing but not much of a problem for medicine and not one at all for management. This ideology of accountability frames two quite different kinds of question: a conventional one (more of the same) and a radical one (enough is enough). Thus the conventional problem of accountability is the problem of moving an echelon of nurses into a quasi-doctoring, semi-biomedical role in the new 'cost-effective' health care system. Meanwhile, health care assistants (or 'aides'), who are assistants to these new nurses, will take on the hierarchical bottom-rung position previously reserved for nursing. The question of their accountability is for the present regarded as largely unproblematic, simply because it is openly recognised that they are *assistants*.[11] The radical problem of accountability is how to make health care, and thus nursing, *publicly* accountable, accountable to sick and injured people, the aged, mothers, disabled people, young people with HIV, children and so on.

THE BROKEN CIRCLE

If we think of how, in general terms, responsibility works out in the health care system we have in the UK what do we find? Nurses in the official view are primarily accountable to patients.[12] But they are not accountable simply as ordinary citizens, in ordinary moral terms, because nursing is one layer in an *institution*. Nursing accountability is moral responsibility narrowed down by the role of nurse. But what a nurse is, is defined by the institution of health care in which she is one element. So the nature of that accountability to patients is moulded by the particular political, economic and administrative form which that institution takes.

This gives rise to a question: where do the moral ends for that accountability come from? What gives the practices of nursing their rightness or wrongness? Ideally, one might suppose, patients should be setting those ends. Nurses should be downwardly accountable. But since nurses work in an institution one has to consider the ends of the institution, professed ends and those which actually emerge in practice. We cannot assume that the ends of the health care institution are the same as the ends set by patients and clients and other people who come into contact with doctors and nurses. Of course, those two sets of ends may overlap, and often do, but sometimes they conflict. (A mother may want to have her baby at home in her own way, but the obstetrician makes a generic warning about 'neonatal risks' and she finds herself in hospital connected to a machine.) The ways in which they conflict may ultimately be more important than the way they overlap. Health care institutions have, besides their professed ends (which make occasional appearances), ends such as income, political power, and prestige and influence.

There are two ways in which the gap between patients' ends and institutional ends are apparently reconciled. One reconciliation takes the form of self-regulation or what may be called lateral accountability. That is, nurses keep a check on each other for the best interests of the patients. The other takes the form of upward accountability. That is, nurses are held in check by the authorities for the best interests of the patients. A little scrutiny reveals these to be ideological in character, that is, tied up with a set of ideas which mask real interests and the real relations of power. The first depends a lot on the notion of honourable, gentlemanly (lady-like) behaviour, which underlies reputation and justifies public trust. The second rests on ideas of authority, the rule of experts, and discipline.

UPWARD ACCOUNTABILITY

Bureaucracies are defined by rules and order, command structures, discipline and rationality. In the manager's mind a lack of accountability means working with employees who are insufficiently subject to sanction, a lack of discipline or liability. One thinks perhaps of an army in which the soldiers do not do as they are told.

The disciplinary understanding of accountability involves looking up the line and doing what the managers and administrators require without question, without challenge (or with only 'suggestion box' lip-service to the freedom to question). All too often in the manager's mind, staff discipline is under threat where there is freedom of thought and action, openness in ideas and decision making, initiative and creativity. Spontaneity is death to bureaucracy. Every bureaucracy requires explicit sanctions to maintain procedures and rules, a system of reporting to superiors and keeping of records to keep every one in line. In the bureaucrat's mind an accountable nurse is one who knows what the procedures are, follows them, and appreciates what the sanctions and penalties are if they are breached.

In a health care system undergoing managerial changes, there have to be changes in administration, that is, in rules and procedures. One must ask: is the present fuss about 'accountability' really all about ensuring that nurses accommodate themselves to a new business-managed health care system?

This kind of accountability inevitably conflicts with morally responsible, or publicly accountable, nursing at many points. In fact, a nurse who takes moral responsibility to patients seriously may be regarded by the powers that be as dangerously unaccountable.

What do managers and administrators regard as 'giving an adequate account' of one's actions? Experience often (but not always) shows that they do not appear to share the moral reactions of front-line health workers and are not much interested in moral justifications for courses of action. They instead seek explanations in terms of 'the facts', and justifications in terms of the set procedures. These facts usually concern matters of human biology and economic cost, and the procedures usually concern matters of administrative convenience and efficiency, and roles and status. Health care bureaucrats are not in a position to give fundamental importance, in their policy decision making, to what patients value in their lives. They operate on the whole on the perfectly understandable premise that patients have no or little power. Health care bureaucracies are run by managers concerned almost entirely with choosing between means, and they take it that the ends are already given by 'society'. But what if society has no voice? If it has no voice one cannot assume that nursing is accountable to the public *by means of* its accountability to the authorities. The circle would be broken.

The first question to be asked, then, is whether modern health care management (and medicine) is able to engage in moral debate. The manager is a crucial 'character' in our society. Alasdair MacIntyre has this to say about this character, and that of 'the therapist' (which we may substitute with 'the doctor'):

> The manager treats ends as given, as outside his scope; his concern is with technique, with effectiveness in transforming raw materials into final products, unskilled labour into skilled labour, investment into profits. The therapist [doctor] also treats ends as given, as outside his scope; his concern also is with technique,

with effectiveness in transforming neurotic symptoms into directed energy, maladjusted individuals into well-adjusted ones. Neither manager nor therapist, in their roles as manager and therapist, do or are able to engage in moral debate.[13]

LATERAL ACCOUNTABILITY

In the mind of the career nurse accountability means autonomous judgement or professional responsibility. To lack accountability here means to be insufficiently independent in judgement and action, not professional, not self-regulatory.

It will be said that it is surely a good thing that nurses are being asked to see themselves as having a clearly defined role, with its own skills, knowledge base, aims and research objectives, and that this role entails specific and distinctive responsibilities which belong to nurses and to no one else. This means that nurses must understand what their distinctive tasks are and what their rationale is, and can no longer regard themselves as the obedient unthinking instruments of doctors and administrators. But what is at stake here?

Accountability as self-regulation is the idea that nurses are accountable to other nurses, for nursing practice, judged by criteria set by nurses. Now, how should this work out in current practice? While no one would wish to deny nurses the standing and rewards they most certainly deserve, let us hope that professional nursing will not even try to model itself on the precedents of the medical and legal occupations. Since the critiques of the late 1960s and early 1970s the very idea of professionalism is questionable. Can we any longer take for granted that it is what the public wants. Certainly, it wants skill and dedication, but does it want an elite which takes self-regulation as an opportunity to protect its own interests, free from public scrutiny?

We know of other professions in which accountability as self-regulation has come to mean little or no public accountability. Ought nursing to model itself on the precedents of the medical and legal occupations? The words of Ivan Illich have even more force today:

> I propose that we name the mid-Twentieth Century 'The Age of Disabling Professions', an age when people had 'problems', experts had 'solutions' and scientists measured imponderables such as 'abilities' and 'needs'. This age is now at an end.[14]

In medicine we find a traditional ideology of 'professional ethics'. The medical profession by its very nature, we are supposed to believe, is dedicated to the public good. A fine ideal. But the ideal and the reality complement one another in an unusual way. The notion of a paternalistic profession dedicated to the public good presupposes that the public does not really recognise its 'best interests' in health matters. Hence the public is largely excluded from health care decision making. The patients' participation is narrowed down to the 'complaints procedure', and even this is treated as merely a vent for 'trouble-makers'. Since the doctor knows best there is no need to involve the patient in health care judgement – such judgements are essentially 'clinical judgements', and economic ones.

The public, I suspect, is increasingly demanding an ethic of deeds rather than an ethic of words. An ethics embedded in patient participation and grass roots public accountability would make professional ethics with its codes and high-sounding exhortations and promises superfluous. What is being said here applies to nursing as well as medicine.

Conflicts of lateral and upward accountability

Lateral accountability and upward accountability come into conflict in a number of ways. A 1989 advisory document produced by the United Kingdom Central Council for Nursing, Midwifery and Health Visiting, and entitled *Exercising Accountability*, gives nurses a professional responsibility for ensuring that informed consent has been obtained. It states that the nurse 'might decide not to co-operate with a procedure if convinced that the decision to agree to it being performed was not truly informed'. The Code recommends that a nurse recall a doctor to give the information again if a discussion with the patient reveals that the doctor has not been understood.[15]

Yet how many concrete steps have been taken by government, health authorities and hospital managers to institute practical procedures and safeguards for nurses who attempt to enact this codified responsibility? Will a nurse who decides 'not to co-operate' be victimised, and what measures can she take if she is? Without safeguards can we really envisage a self-regulating nursing environment in which nurses encourage each other to intervene in cases of invalid consent and take to task those who do not intervene?

A system in crisis poses conflicting necessities: it needs to extend the responsibilities of nurses, but it also needs to do so without threatening the existing power bases. The very thought of empowering half a million UK nurses must disturb some medical technocrats and civil servants. One suspects that many of them would approve of self-regulating nursing so long as it is strictly organised on managerial terms. Without democratic managerial and administrative reforms nursing self-regulation will turn out to be an arm of the existing hierarchy.

DOWNWARD ACCOUNTABILITY

Imagine a 4-year-old, Mary, dying of cancer.[16] After several months of visits to hospital for treatment everyone involved feels that the present admission will be her last. The prognosis is hopeless. The mother has prepared her child for death. Mary, now very weak and thin, is pleased with a story her mother told her in reply to her questions about what death is like:

> You know what it's like when you fall asleep on the armchair and I pick you up and carry you up to your bed, and you don't know anything about it? Well, dying is like that, only this time God will pick you up and take care of you for ever.

In the middle of one night, the newly registered nurse on duty (Joanne) suggests to the exhausted mother that she take a nap in the rest room. A little later Mary awakes, struggling to breathe and looking very frightened. Joanne calls the other staff and asks for the mother to be brought in. There is a delay. Joanne, remembering the story the mother had told Mary, picks up the child and sits gently rocking her in her arms. Mary calms down and dies peacefully holding the nurse's hand.

Joanne is still sitting there when the doctor arrives and begins to reprimand her for not taking steps to resuscitate Mary. The nurse tries to justify her action, saying that the child was dying and the important thing was that she die in peace. 'How dare you behave as though you are not accountable to anyone!' the consultant demands.

Later the nurse is summoned to a disciplinary hearing. She is reminded that she must be 'accountable' at all times and that all patients should be resuscitated unless an explicit medical decision to the contrary has been made. Joanne points out that she had understood that the doctor had verbally advised the senior nurse that Mary should not be resuscitated, but nothing was in writing, there had been no case conference, no multidisciplinary discussion, and the nurses had not been consulted. Personally, she could not understand why the child had not been allowed to die at home, she said politely.

Joanne is coldly told that the incident will be put in her personal record, she is warned, given a lecture the main theme of which is that she is 'only a nurse' and then 'let off'. As she walks back to the ward she remembers Mary and in her heart she feels she had done the right thing. Something is wrong with the institution, she suspects. For a few days she toys with the idea of leaving nursing and seeking work with greater freedom, in a bank for example. Under the daily pressure of work she has no further chance to think about the meaning of what has happened, let alone discuss the matter with others. From now on she is more cautious. For the institution, she has become a 'better' nurse. In truth she has begun to apply the brakes on caring.

Some readers will not find this story typical of what happens in their own institution. But they may be able to think of other situations similar in essential respects. It represents the kind of situation which countless nurses find themselves in every day, situations in which their moral sense is subverted by the mindless demands and constraints of the institution in which they work.

This nurse understood her 'accountability' in quite immediate terms. If she had thought about it at all she might have spoken of her moral responsibility to the child and the child's mother. In terms of her role as a nurse one might say she was acting with downward accountability. In fact, speaking of 'accountability' here is strained and probably inappropriate – she simply did what she knew to be right. However, if asked by management to 'give an account' of her action then simply replying that she 'knew it to be right' would not suffice. Hospital management understands accountability quite differently, and this is the conception that prevails. She had failed to see that she 'had a job to do', and that job was not defined by her but by the institution.

Conflicts of downward and upward accountability

What we have in this story is a case of a more general problem – a conflict of downward and upward accountability. Professionally, and in nurse education, nurses are presented as being directly and primarily accountable to their patients. Naturally, one might think this had something to do with kindness, patience and understanding for example. In reality they are only very indirectly accountable to patients by being directly and primarily accountable to the management (nursing, medical and financial). But one might speculate that there would be a kind of circle of accountability if the management set the rules in accordance with what it takes to be in the public's best interests. Nurses, we are asked to believe, do not really know. In other words, downward accountability is expressed *through* upward accountability, in which the medical/economic management is the proxy for the public. Expressed in this way it is distorted by the self-serving interests of the health care establishment, but perhaps (one imagines) this could be mitigated in various ways.

Unfortunately, as I had suggested earlier, the problem may be deeper than it appears at first sight. For, as I asked earlier, are managers (or anyone else) *able* to represent the public? Just as problematic: can *any* institution be a vehicle for virtues such as kindness, patience, understanding and generosity?

Let us approach this in terms of a common experience. Everyone who works in health care is aware of what one may call an Inverse Square Law of Accountability: the more important the decision making the less contact the decision makers have with those affected by the decisions. The closer the health carer is to the patient or client the less freedom and power that health carer has, as a general rule. Midwifery and community nursing, which have traditionally had a high degree of autonomy, have also become subject to this law of bureaucratic hierarchy. The greater the distance of the decision maker the more emphasis is put on grandiloquent and solemn pledges of 'dedicated service', 'utmost respect for human life' and 'conscience and dignity' by way of verbal compensation.

If we open our eyes for a moment and admit that the medical management does not in fact know what is in the interests of patients (although they know quite a bit about how human bodies work) and the economic management does not in fact know what serves public welfare (although they are – let us allow – expert at cost-effectiveness), then we may wonder whether health care management serves, or can serve, any moral end whatsoever.

The conflict between downward and upward accountability is generally evident in the ordinary assessments which ordinary people make of health care professionals. A parent of a Down's Syndrome child says of parents such as himself:

> I don't think you can fairly compare us with professionals. How can you be equal, you can't be *equal*. You both know different things, you're both responsible for different aspects. I mean parents, in my eyes, parents are responsible for their children, totally; professionals are employed to do their job.[17]

Corporate accountability

In some contexts to lack accountability means to act in an arbitrary or capricious fashion. It also means acting autocratically, without checks and balances. Nicolae Ceausescu of Romania lacked accountability in this sense. Here the concept of 'accountability' is closely allied with that of democracy.

I maintain that the real issue of health care in Europe is not so much the accountability of individual nurses, midwives and health visitors, but the accountability of the health care authorities – administrators, managers (including nurse managers), health authorities, Trust managers, medical consultants, research bodies, civil servants and government.

In the 1991–2 scandal involving the Bank of Credit and Commerce International (BCCI) one investigator said publicly: 'The big people were getting away with things the little guy wouldn't imagine he could get away with.' We ought perhaps to ask whether the same is true in health care. How often are managers, administrators or medical consultants made to give an account? Are we really to believe that somehow they are more virtuous and public spirited than the rest of us?

The truth is that at present very few mechanisms exist, at least in the UK, to hold a health authority to account for acting without proper regard for the public welfare. Those that do exist have hardly been tested.

The current UK 'market reforms' have made matters worse rather than better. Accountability for a health authority or trust hospital is now increasingly seen only as a matter of the efficient cost-cutting use of resources. The UK government's 'White Paper' on the reforms explicitly proposed to eliminate representation by the public, trade unions and local authorities and emphasised business management with upward accountability through a strong chain of command and this proposal has now been effected.[18]

At present, says the Paper, District Health Authorities (DHAs) 'are neither truly representative nor management bodies'. To avoid this supposed 'confusion' they are made entirely managerial. The same goes for the authorities' Family Practitioner Committees (FPCs).[19] It might occur to the rest of us that the supposed confusion could equally well have been resolved by making them entirely representative – but that would have been democratic.

What about the patients' representative bodies, the Community Health Councils (CHCs)? The Paper says that CHCs will act as 'a channel for consumer views to health authorities and FPCs', but no proposals have been made for strengthening them and presumably they will be merely advisory and rather powerless.[20] The FPC's sub-committees on patients' complaints will still be needed, we are told, but no recommendations are made to ensure public accountability.

It is striking that the Paper is prescriptive, and directive in tone, in its business management proposals, but merely tentative and suppositional in its proposals for dealing with patient complaints and injustices. Thus:

> To make sure that patients' personal as well as clinical needs are being met, health authorities will *wish* to monitor patient satis-faction, *perhaps* through the systematic use of questionnaires and follow-up surveys. As a quality control measure, contracts *could* require the hospital to provide reports on all complaints received and the action taken to remedy them.[21]

Regarding the new self-governing hospitals (Trusts, which run their own budgets and provide contractual services to Health Author-ities): 'It will therefore be for each Trust to determine whether it wishes to open its routine meetings to the public or Community Health Council representatives.'[22]

The corporate accountability of the authorities certainly stands in urgent need of honest reappraisal; and one might have expected nursing to play a great part in this. However, in nursing a corporate identity and responsibility has hardly arisen at all. Exhortations to *individual* 'accountability' on the part of nurses are now com-monplace, although (as I have argued) institutional structures and ideology make this almost impossible for an individual nurse to effect. Meanwhile the *corporate* ethical responsibility of nursing does not appear on any significant agenda. Indeed, if it did, then radical questions would have to be asked about the background assumptions of nursing itself, most notably its subordination.

Salvage has correctly noted how nursing accountability is nearly always cast in the context of individualism. That is, nursing accountability is thought to be about the individual nurse being answerable to the individual patient. The 'named nurse' initiative (under the Patients' Charter) continues a development which began with the Nursing Process.

> This stress on individual responsibility while in some ways being welcome also neglects the role and possibility of acting together – suddenly, despite being part of the profession, you're on your own.[23]

The questions of why nursing has hardly developed a corporate identity and hardly engages in collective action are ones which strike at the very roots of its ethical status.[24]

A savage inquiry

As an illustration of my points about managerial accountability it is useful to recall the familiar case of Dr Wendy Savage. She was the obstetrician who was suspended in April 1985 from her work at The London Hospital until a public inquiry into her competence completely exonerated her. (The inquiry took place in February 1986.) The issue was that Dr Savage thought she should allow mothers control over their own childbirth. That was her understanding of accountability. In her book she asks:

> How is it possible that the Chairman of the Health Authority and a handful of doctors could set in motion an enquiry costing an estimated £250,000 at a time when the impoverished district of Tower Hamlets is cutting beds and services? To whom is the Chairman of the DHA accountable? To the people of Tower Hamlets? To the Government? To the Regional Health Authority?[25]

Although over 100 Members of Parliament called for the resignation of the Chairman, according to Savage he expressed no regrets at the time about his actions. Savage concludes: 'The whole system seems to lack any mechanism for assessing the performance of a Health Authority except in one way – can they keep within their budget?'[26]

There is now a great interest in the law in nurse education. Managers are usually quite prepared to send nurses on law courses to enhance their 'accountability'. This is all very well, for nurses should be acquainted with the law of negligence, health and safety, trespass to the person and so on. But this is more upward accountability, more defensiveness. The patient is seen as a potential trouble-maker and threat to the interests of the health authorities and Trusts rather than their *raison d'être*.

Nurses in fact need to have knowledge of the law to defend themselves not against patients but against managers, administrators, consultants, health authorities and even the government. Of special importance perhaps are employment law and European laws on civil rights.

There is no doubt in my mind that nursing cannot make progress without dealing with the issue of non-accountable bureaucracy, whether public sector or private. Nurses, like many other employees in our society, are constrained to behave as passive participants in an impersonal 'rationalised' machine. Much sociological evidence has accumulated to show, and everyday experience confirms, that specialisation, hierarchy and professionalisation in the health labour force serve to consolidate the power of the economic and political Establishment and disempower the needy.[27]

COMPLETING THE CIRCLE

One could adopt two responses to this situation, a utopian one and a compromise. The utopian response is to take away power from doctors and make them technical advisers to nurses, midwives and health visitors (in the way laboratory technicians have no power but only technical expertise); and to take power away from managers, fundamentally decentralising and democratising the health service beyond anything we have even imagined so far, and making nurses responsive within small-scale health care set-ups to the health care representatives of the community.

There are many compromise responses. They all begin with piecemeal legislative changes to bring management nearer to identifying with the best interests of the public. The idea is that if management can be made accountable to the public then any nurse would be downwardly accountable in the very act of being upwardly accountable. To put it simply: if the nurse is meant to serve the patient then as long as the manager really is accountable to the patient then the nurse will be doing the right thing simply in doing whatever the manager says. We might think of this as a kind of informed paternalism. I wonder whether this is not even more utopian than the first solution offered!

As examples of the kind of piecemeal legislative changes which may advance public accountability, the following are worthy of consideration: local council elections should include election of health authority members (and nurses should be encouraged to stand); Community Health Councils should be reorganised as independent investigative and monitoring bodies with powers supported by the law; health authorities should have a publicly available constitution which sets out aims, limits on power, user rights, explicit complaints procedures etc.; annual and publicly accessible reports should be prepared by each provider unit (hospital, family doctor, etc.) on positive steps taken to ensure public accountability, including exactly how complaints have been remedied; the law enabling access to the meetings of public bodies should be enforced and widened so that the public has access to the major administrative meetings of all hospitals, and other health care units; the General Medical Council, which registers doctors, ought to be reformed to make it thoroughly accountable to the public and individual complainants;[28] there should be statutory protection for employees who 'blow the whistle' on unacceptable practices; there should be a Freedom of Information Act to give the public access to health care information and decisions.

The law in itself will not bring about the necessary changes. Nurses and other health carers should be taking new initiatives in linking up with patient groups to find mechanisms of public accountability: patient's committees, members' groups at day centres, health councils, and so on.[29] Above all, a change in attitudes and culture is necessary.

Decent health care, and the future of nursing, depends on closing the circle of accountability.

NOTES

1 Salvage, J., *The Politics of Nursing*, London: Heinemann, 1985, p. 2.
2 Pyne, R., *Professional Discipline in Nursing, Midwifery and Health Visiting*, Oxford: Blackwell Scientific, 2nd edn, 1992, p. 23.
3 On how a 'mediated' profession contrasts with 'collegiate' and 'patronage' professions see Hugman, R., *Power in Caring Professions*, London: Macmillan, 1991, pp. 3–4.
4 See Savage, J., *Nurses, Gender and Sexuality*, London: Heinemann, 1987; Holmes, H.B. and Purdy, L.M. (eds), *Feminist Perspectives in Medical Ethics*, Indiana, Indiana University Press, 1992.

5 This article draws on my earlier articles, in *Nursing Standard*, 1991, vol. 6 (4), pp. 49–50; 1992, vol. 6 (15), pp. 46–7; 1992, vol. 6 (21), pp. 44–5 and a presentation at the 1992 European Congress of Nursing (Amsterdam), subsequently published in *Vakblad voor verpleegkundigen*, 1992, vol. 19, pp. 677–82. Some earlier discussions of accountability in nursing are: Royal College of Nursing, *Accountability in Nursing*, London: RCN, 1980; Bergman, R., 'Accountability: Definitions and Dimensions', *International Nursing Review*, 1981, vol. 28 (2), pp. 53–9; Millard, R., 'The New Accountability', *Nursing Outlook*, 1975, vol. 23 (8), pp. 496–500.

6 For an analysis of nursing in terms of Max Weber's category of rationality see Hewa, S. and Hetherington, R.W., 'Specialists without Spirit: Crisis in the Nursing Profession', *Journal of Medical Ethics*, 1990, vol. 16, pp. 179–84.

7 For more on the expanding role of the nurse in relation to science and technique see Hunt, G. and Wainwright, P. (eds), *Expanding the Role of the Nurse*, Oxford: Blackwell Scientific, 1994.

8 See for example the statement about the centrality of obedience in Dock, S., 'The Relation of the Nurse to the Doctor and the Doctor to the Nurse', *American Journal of Nursing*, 1917, vol. 17, p. 394.

9 The recent General Medical Council's performance procedures may take doctors's public accountability further while, I suspect, primarily bringing medicine into line with the technical demands of the new economic management of health care. See General Medical Council, *Proposals for New Performance Procedures: A Consultation Paper*, London: GMC, May 1992.

10 Goodey, C.F. (ed.), *Living in the Real World: Families Speak about Down's Syndrome*, London: The Twenty-One Press, 1991, p. 102.

11 See Hunt, G., 'Project 2000 – Ethics, Ambivalence and Ideology', in O. Slevin and M. Buckenham (eds), *Project 2000: The Teachers Speak*, Edinburgh: Campion Press, 1992, especially pp. 97–8.

12 One finds a statement about the 'primacy of the interests of patients or clients' and about patient 'advocacy' in United Kingdom Central Council, *Exercising Accountability*, London: UKCC, 1989.

13 MacIntyre, A., *After Virtue: A Study in Moral Theory*, London: Duckworth, 2nd edn, 1985, p. 30.

14 Illich, I., *Disabling Professions*, London: Marion Boyars, 1987, p. 11.

15 United Kingdom Central Council, op. cit., Sec.D.

16 Adapted, and combined with some personal anecdotes, from a story in Curtin, L. and Flaherty, M. J. (eds), *Nursing Ethics: Theories and Pragmatics*, Englewood Cliffs, N.J: Prentice-Hall, 1982, pp. 293–4.

17 Goodey, op. cit., p. 98.

18 See Hunt, G., '"Patient Choice" and the National Health Service Review', *Journal of Social Welfare Law*, 1990, vol. 4, pp. 245–55.

19 Department of Health, *Working for Patients*, (CM555), London: Department of Health, 1989 (and eight Working Papers), paras. 8.3–8.7, 7.23–7.29.

20 Department of Health, op. cit., para. 8.7.

21 Department of Health, op. cit., *Working Paper* 1, para. 2.13, emphasis mine.

22 Department of Health, op. cit., *Working Paper* 1, para. 3.7.
23 Salvage, op. cit., pp. 98–9.
24 On the political history of nursing two recent useful books are: Owens,
    P. and Glennerster, H. (eds), *Nursing in Conflict*, London: Macmillan,
    1990; Holden P. and Littlewood, J. (eds), *Anthropology and Nursing*,
    London: Routledge, 1991.
25 Savage, W., *A Savage Inquiry: Who Controls Childbirth?* London:
    Virago, 1986, p. 178.
26 ibid.
27 See Turner, B.S., *Medical Power and Social Knowledge*, London: Sage,
    1987.
28 Robinson, J., *A Patient Voice at the GMC: A Lay Member's View of the
    General Medical Council*, London: Health Rights, 1988.
29 See Croft, S. and Beresford, P., 'User Involvement, Citizenship and
    Social Policy', *Critical Social Policy*, 1989, vol. 26, pp. 5–18.

Chapter 8

The value of codes of conduct

Andrew Edgar

This chapter seeks to explore the purpose, nature and limitations of the nurses' code of conduct. It will be argued that the interpretation and application of any code of conduct rests upon the informal moral beliefs and social skills of the profession's practitioners. While these beliefs and skills are a necessary resource upon which the profession must draw, they may also present a threat to the stability of the profession. Codes of conduct are formulated in such a manner as to manage the resultant tension between the formal and informal norms of the profession. The nurses' code will be assessed in terms of its response to this tension, through comparison with other professional codes.[1]

The *Code of Professional Conduct*, drawn up by the United Kingdom Central Council for Nursing, Midwifery and Health Visiting (UKCC), was first published in 1983, and revised in 1984 and 1992. Its structure is typical of such codes, being that of a short preamble, emphasising the behaviour expected of the practitioner, followed by a set of principles governing specific aspects of conduct. In virtually all codes, the generality of such principles entails the development of some form of annotation. The Code is now complemented by a series of advisory papers (including *Advertising*, *Confidentiality*, *Administration of Medicines*, and *Exercising Accountability* and a document about removal from the register).[2]

UNDERPINNINGS

A general criticism put against codes of conduct is that they are the unargued presentation of the dos and don'ts of the profession.[3] They lack any coherent underpinning in terms of normative ethics, and as such amount to the reification of a more or less arbitrary series of moral intuitions.

This may be illustrated by reference to paragraph 7 of the UKCC's Code, that requires the practitioner to 'recognise and respect the uniqueness and dignity of each patient and client, and respond to their need for care, irrespective of their ethnic origin, religious beliefs'. While such a principle is important, it provides no guidance as to how conflicts between professional beliefs and the client's beliefs are to be resolved. In the code of the British Association of Social Workers (BASW), the annotation to paragraph 10.4 reads: 'it is sometimes necessary to help the client to abandon pseudo- or fantasy-choices so that effective choices may be made'.

While an ethics of respect may be defended, the extreme suggested by Harris, such that the autonomy of patients involves the 'freedom to make irrational or capricious choices, if that is what [they wish] to do' makes no allowance for beliefs that may entail law breaking (such as the desire for active euthanasia) or beliefs that, if realised as actions, would harm others.[4]

However, the purpose of this chapter is not to defend the development of coherent normative ethics to underpin such codes. It is rather to recognise and assess the effective grounding that the codes already have in the practitioners' informal beliefs.

INCOMPLETENESS

This analysis can be developed by noting that any practice-governing rule is necessarily incomplete in itself. Its precise application to a given situation, and hence its meaning, must be governed by an infinite series of additional rules. As Wieder has noted, the interpretation of an utterance depends upon,

(a) who was saying it . . . ; (b) to whom it was being said . . . ; (c) where it was being said . . . ; (d) on what kind of occasion it was being said . . . ; (e) the social relationship between teller and hearer . . . ; and so forth.[5]

While a code of conduct is designed to be applicable to a more diffuse set of social situations than, say, an utterance made in face-to-face conversation, assumptions about the authors of the code, the audience, the power relationship between the two, and so forth, will be implicit in any interpretation of the code.

The interpretation of a rule-governing principle, and hence the repair of its indexical nature, will rest upon the life world presupposed by the interpreter. The concept of 'life world' was originally proposed by Husserl and Schutz, and most recently revitalized by Habermas.[6] It refers to the skills and experiences that the member of the community requires in order to act effectively in the (social and natural) world. Schutz and Luckmann define the life world as 'the unexamined ground of everything given in my experience . . . the taken-for-granted frame in which all the problems which I must overcome are placed'.[7] The problem of interpreting and applying a principle from a code of conduct is resolved by (more or less unreflective) appeal to specific competences held by the professional. The competent social actor will have the skill, when confronted by a novel situation, to relate it to specific known, and unproblematic, types, and thus if relevant, to the code. This may be illustrated in more detail.

The main principles of a code tend to be so general as to become trivial. The indexical nature of a code is partially repaired by its annotations. The Royal Pharmaceutical Society's code's paragraph 1 may illustrate this: 'A pharmacist's prime concern shall be for the welfare of both patients and public.' The annotations to this principle list a series of situations that may provide problems to the pharmacist, and of which the code serves to make them aware. These include the sale of slimming and other non-medical products, sale of chemicals, and sales by post. Such annotations amount to a catalogue of the problems that have confronted pharmacists, and for which they may be expected to take responsibility. The professional is being warned not to take certain situations for granted. It may then be suggested that in the repairing of the indexicality of a code the presupposition of a coherent normative ethics is of less (or indeed of no) importance in comparison with the collective practical experience of the profession.

However, if a principle is necessarily incomplete, then so too are its annotations. While the above example indicates the importance of annotations (and a weakness of the UKCC's Code is the lack of a comprehensive set of annotations, or even readily accessible 'case law' as to the principles' application[8]), ultimately appeal must be made to the informal rules acknowledged within the profession, and within everyday social practice.

Paragraph 1.6 of the pharmaceutical code, ruling on the excessive consumption of laxatives for slimming purposes, notes that the pharmacist should 'refuse sales if there is reason to believe such products are being misused'. This rests upon two presuppositions. First, there is no explanation of why such use of laxatives is 'misuse'. That the explanation is obvious demonstrates the appeal to a taken-for-granted set of beliefs that is part of the substantive life world of most (but by no means all) members of contemporary British society. Second, no further criteria are given by which such misuse could be judged at the point of purchase. Again, any attempt to explicate such criteria, being beyond simple quantification, would be in vain. The skills of the pharmacist as a competent member of society will, in general, be adequate to the task.

THE HIDDEN CURRICULUM

This repairing of the indexicality of a code through appeal to the life world raises further problems. It may be accepted that all members of a society will not necessarily have the same substantive understanding of the life world. Hence, even professionals may bring different competences to the problem of interpreting and applying a code. Professional training to some degree mitigates against this. The extensive training undergone by the professional entails both the mastery of an overt curriculum of relevant technical skills and knowledges, and a hidden curriculum of professional norms and values. It may be suggested that the hidden curriculum grounds a professional life world. Because all members of the profession have passed through a similar education, the individual members' perception of the professional life world will be more unified than is the case with the pre-professional life world.

The professional is effectively sundered from the more diffuse beliefs and skills of the pre-professional. A potential conflict between the professional and non-professional may continue to exist, and become explicit through the use of pre- or non-professional moral beliefs as a resource to challenge professional morality.

An extreme example, that illustrates the conflict that can exist between lay and professional interpretation of codes, has been documented by Glazer.[9] In the case of the American police force, a tension exists between the ideals seemingly espoused in its code, and actual practice. The formulation of the code of conduct conforms to the expectations of lay morality, and yet is not generally followed within the force. New recruits must therefore learn to subordinate their lay understanding and implementation of the code to its actual, professional abuse. (In effect, the professional life world recognises an important caveat for interpreting the code: these rules are not to be taken seriously.)

With reference to nursing, Heywood Jones makes what may be a corroborating point, by noting that those with the least experience of organisational structures are the most likely to be whistleblowers.[10]

At a more typical level, conflict occurs between members of a profession, not over the question of whether a code should be taken seriously at all, but over precise applications. A disunity may occur through the existence of competing versions of the professional life world itself, as norms and values inherent to the professional life world are disputed. A code's function within the profession's disciplinary procedures highlights this.

SELF-REGULATION

The Nurses, Midwives and Health Visitors Act 1979, provided for the formation of the UKCC (alongside the four national boards), with its primary function of establishing and improving standards of training and professional conduct. The nursing profession has the legal status of a protected monopoly. This may be seen as a key element in the reinforcing of the professional status of British nursing. A profession will have a governing body, free of external interference, that controls admission to the profession, and may expel members from the profession. The legal protection of clients is thereby devolved onto this governing body.[11]

The code is central to the self-regulatory mechanisms of a profession. In the case of the UKCC, the *Code of Professional Conduct* serves as a set of criteria, against which allegations of misconduct may be assessed. The UKCC's document, 'with a view to removal from the register', notes that someone with a potential complaint against a nurse should be aware that the Code is one of the items that the Professional Conduct Committee will have in mind in assessing allegations.[12] In disciplining a member, an option open to the national boards or to the Professional Conduct Committee is for no action to be taken other than advice referring to the relevant sections of the Code.[13] Hence, a code of conduct is an integral part of the response that a profession can make to allegations, from colleagues, clients or the general public, against members.[14]

Yet a profession's interest in its code is disputed. The analysis of professionalisation has polarised between those that took the high rewards and power of the professions to reflect, and depend upon, their actual utility (or function) to society, and those that held that such rewards and power result from the manipulation of the image of professional utility.[15] This may be presented, in outline, in terms of a dichotomy between trust and legitimacy.

Codes themselves may insist upon the trust that the client must have in the profession, and that high standards of professional conduct are integral to the maintenance of such trust. The Royal Pharmaceutical Society code notes, in paragraph 2, that a 'pharmacist shall uphold the honour and dignity of the profession and not engage in any activity which may bring the profession into disrepute'. The UKCC requires that the practitioner should 'act, at all times, in such a manner as to . . . justify public trust and confidence'. Taken at face value, such claims may be interpreted as merely emphasising that, if the profession is to continue to provide its particular service, and therefore continue to be of value to society as a whole, then the trust of the clients and wider public is a necessary precondition that should be promoted and protected. The [American] National Association of Social Workers' code (paragraph V.M.1) brilliantly, but perversely perhaps, demands that the 'social worker should protect and enhance the dignity and integrity of the profession and should be responsible and vigorous in discussion and criticism of the profession'.

The counter-argument is to claim that codes and internal disciplinary procedures serve to legitimate the privileges and autonomy of the profession. A tension exists between 'trust' and 'legitimacy' in so far as the former may be taken to entail an attitude that is grounded in an objective understanding of the profession's qualities, and the latter implies some process of manipulation of public and client perception such that undesirable qualities are concealed or reinterpreted. In this context Kultgen writes of 'The Ideological Use of Professional Codes'.[16] McKinlay has argued that codes are 'political counters constructed as much to serve as public evidence of professional intentions and ideals as to provide actual behavioural guidelines for practitioners'.[17]

WHISTLEBLOWING

Cases of whistleblowing tend to highlight clearly the relationship of a code to the internal power structures of the profession. Paragraph 11 of the UKCC's Code might be thought by an outsider to approve of whistleblowing, affirming that the practitioner should 'report to an appropriate person or authority . . . any circumstances in the environment of care which could jeopardise standards of practice'. However, the phrase 'appropriate person or authority' requires knowledge of the professional life world in order to be interpreted with any precision.[18] The UKCC's *Exercising Accountability* glosses this, as if it were unproblematic, as the 'immediate professional manager'.[19] This is quite unexceptional. Indeed, it clarifies much of the ambiguity of the original principle.

As Kultgen has shown, the phrasing of the National [American] Society of Professional Engineers' code has led to conflict over exactly what other authorities may be appropriate.[20] Yet the UKCC gloss entails that conflicts must be resolved within the profession, and indeed within the formal management hierarchy. This suggests that statements to the press, for example, however grave the problem, or however reluctant to respond the professional hierarchy may be, are generally unacceptable.

From a critical perspective, codes of conduct may therefore be seen to *insulate*, more or less explicitly, the profession from the criticisms of the ambient society. If the non-professional life world does indeed offer a resource by which criticisms of the profession may be developed and sustained, then it is in a conservative profession's interest to insulate itself from this resource. Disputes are typically to be resolved internally, without external knowledge or interference. This extends and legitimates the legal monopoly. Public morality is not allowed to violate professional morality at an institutional level.[21]

INSULATION

This process of insulation from public morality may be seen in another of its aspects in the code of the Royal Pharmaceutical Society (RPS). Paragraph 2.2 notes that a pharmacist should not use '"Doctor" or "Dr" on the fascia of a retail pharmacy business or on dispensing labels' because it would be misleading. The taken-for-granted assumptions of the lay member of society include the equation of 'doctor' with a medical doctor. This could indeed, in the case of pharmacy, lead to potentially serious misunderstandings. Paragraph sixteen of the UKCC's Code, relating to advertising, may be seen to rest equally, and not unfairly, upon assumptions concerning lay misunderstandings.

A similar appeal is made to the non-professional life world when the RPS code asserts that, 'Exhibition of merchandise and dumper bins outside pharmacy premises is unprofessional. Anyone seeking to use trestle boards outside premises should recognise the need for the environs of the premises to reflect the professional nature of pharmacy' (para. 8.3). Again, the potential for the non-professional to misunderstand a situation is emphasised. Yet here the situation is seemingly more trivial. Within a critical perspective, it may be suggested that the confusion is at root one between a professional and a shopkeeper, risking the consequent loss of status of the professional. In both of these examples the beliefs and skills embodied in the non-professional life world are disparaged in favour of the professional competence.

The process of insulation may be seen in a final aspect by further reference to paragraph six of the second edition of the UKCC's Code (rephrased in paragraph seven of the third edition). In its exhortation to 'Take account of the customs, values and spiritual beliefs of patients/clients', it serves to devalue the beliefs held by the practitioner. This suggests the impoverishment of the practitioners' own lives.[22] The personal attributes of the practitioner are encoded as a hindrance, rather than a resource. This encoding may take a number of forms. The American Medical Association's code emphasises the responsibility to 'expose those physicians deficient in character or competence' (paragraph II). The 1953 code of the International Council of Nurses notes that the 'nurse in private life adheres to standards of personal ethics which reflect credit upon [the] profession' (paragraph 12). (There is no parallel principle in the 1973 code.)

In this context, the UKCC's Code demands in paragraph eight that the practitioner should 'report to an appropriate person or authority, at the earliest possible time, any conscientious objection which may be relevant to your professional practice'. The principle's negative tone may be highlighted by considering a positive reading: the practitioner should make known to an appropriate person or authority any moral wisdom or personal qualities and experience which may be relevant to professional practice. In any case, paragraph eight adds little. Conscientious objection to involvement in abortion is already protected by section four of the 1967 Abortion Act (so exists independently of the UKCC's statement). *Exercising Accountability* glosses the principle, making reference to 'resuscitative treatment of the elderly, the transfusion of blood, or electroconvulsive therapy', but only to state that the practitioner 'must make their position clear to their professional colleagues and managers, *and recognise that this may have implications for their contract of employment*'.[23]

RESPONSIBILITY

Underlying this dichotomising of professional and non-professional life worlds is a specific characterisation of the professional practitioner. Such characterisation rests upon the ultimate responsibility (or accountability) of the professional for their actions. It is this that allows the equating of codes of professional conduct with codes of ethics. The ethical nature of any code is justified in terms of the centrality of responsibility.

The BASW code states that the 'assumption of personal responsibility for one's work is crucial to professionalism. A completely bureaucratised service cannot be a professional one' (annotation to principle seven). The Royal Pharmaceutical Society's code notes under the title 'Professional Responsibility' (paragraph 3.4) that, 'As an independent practitioner a pharmacist should act within his professional competence and be personally responsible for his decisions.'

The UKCC's *Administration of Medicines* defines 'professional judgement in health care' as 'personal judgement based on special knowledge and skill', adding later that the exercise of professional judgement 'will lead the practitioner to satisfy himself/herself that he/she is competent to administer the medicine and prepared to be accountable for that action'.[24] While the UKCC is near to an explicit acknowledgement of the non-professional life world, the use of 'personal responsibility' in all these cases emphasises that, as a professional, the practitioner can look to no one else to take the blame for failures.

This may be systematised, somewhat crudely, by suggesting a tripartite classification of life worlds that underpins professional codes, as a presupposition to their interpretation in accord with the expectations of professional regulatory bodies. This is a hierarchy of professional, pre-professional and non-professional life worlds, such that the professional life world (learned as the hidden curriculum of training and further developed through professional experience) is of most relevance to interpretation in professional life.

The pre-professional life world would include a more diffuse set of beliefs and competencies, held by the bulk of practitioners before training, and continuing as the basis of their off-duty, 'private' moral sense. This may further be identified as a class culture, in that it would broadly correspond to the set of beliefs and competences held by the professional classes. This is to suggest that such a set exists, and that any given profession will draw upon this set, thematising and developing certain of its elements in its professional life world. The pre-professional life world contains the roots of professional responsibility in less well defined, and less rigorously sanctioned, normative models of personal competence and autonomy. It is at this level that the UKCC's 'personal judgement' occurs.

From the perspective of the professional life world, the non-professional (which is to say, the member of a class or status group that diverges markedly from the professional group) is deemed as being of minimal competence. In effect, the competences that the non-professional does have are deemed irrelevant by the standards of the professional life world. Such competences can never form the basis for professionalism. They may lead to the misunderstanding of the word 'doctor', or the making of 'pseudo- and fantasy-choices', for example. In implicitly identifying a non-professional life world, the profession legitimates its protection of those clients and members of the public that have only this competence, albeit at the risk of paternalism. (Implicit to this classification is the tension between legitimacy and trust, which is to say between the benign and critical views of professionalism. This is discussed further below.)

The criticism of the tendency of codes of conduct to sunder professional and lay life worlds cannot assume that the lay life world is always necessarily supportive of the code and integral to its moral interpretation. The National Association of Social Workers' code notes both that the 'ethical behaviour of social workers results not from edict, but from a personal commitment of the individual', and that the 'private conduct of the social worker is a personal matter to the same degree as is any other person's, except when such conduct compromises the fulfilment of professional responsibilities'.[25] Here the tension of private and professional belief is intuited, and managed in the text through the separation of 'personal commitment' from the 'personal matter' of 'private conduct'. The precise difference in content, if any, is thereby intimated rather than explicated by a difference in wording.

The UKCC manages this in a similarly *ad hoc* and at times oblique manner (as has been suggested with reference to paragraph seven of the Code). Section G of *Exercising Accountability* recognises the potential tension of the beliefs commonly held by non-practitioners to those (that are ideally) held by practitioners. It is emphasised that a practitioner's refusal to be associated 'with patients suffering from Hepatitis B Infection and those with Acquired Immune Deficiency Syndrome' can find no support in the Code.

Examples of prejudice highlight the point that the relationship between the private and professional beliefs of the practitioner must be scrutinized. At present, the only UKCC statement against prejudice is this passage, concluding with the assertion that the 'UKCC expects its practitioners to adopt a non-judgemental approach in the exercise of their caring role'.[26]

BASW's code contains the following principle of practice: the social worker 'will not act selectively towards clients out of prejudice on the grounds of their origin, status, sex, sexual orientation, age, belief or contribution to society' (paragraph 10.3). The formulation is particularly neat, and is reinforced by an annotation that recognises that 'no one is entirely free from prejudices'. This is developed, in paragraph 10.6, to the effect that the social worker 'will give precedence to [their] professional responsibility over [their] personal interests', which, in turn, is annotated to note that the principle 'does not imply that at all times the social worker must put [their] responsibility to a client above [their] other responsibilities, for example, as a citizen or as a parent'.

Situations in which clients or the public do misunderstand technical concepts, or make choices that may be deemed to be fantastic, further highlight the problematic relationship between the professional and non-professional life worlds. BASW's annotation to paragraph 10.4, makes an implicit appeal to the complex skills that the social worker will have developed to identify fantasy-choices. It is not a code's purpose to detail such skills, even if that were possible. The code rather rests upon these professional, as opposed to non- or pre-professional skills. However, the danger remains that the client's competence may be totally undermined, and the profession may thereby further insulate itself from its professed purpose. Acceptance that the client's choices may not be fantasies, or at least acceptance of the need to establish why the non-professional life world diverges so markedly from the professional, may be necessary to overcome both individual and institutional prejudice.

Section E of the UKCC's *Exercising Accountability* makes a very cautious response to this problem, appealing to the practitioner's 'exercise of judgement', but emphasising that the right of decision should be taken away from the patient or relatives only 'in the rarest of cases'.[27]

PROFESSIONALISATION

In the above account, it has been argued that a critical perspective on the professions throws some light upon the use of their codes, and the presuppositions in which those codes are embedded. Yet the position of what has been called the 'lower' professions, including social work and nursing, is more complex than the critical perspective would allow. The critical perspective was developed in response to the so-called higher professions. The professional status of nursing is, in contrast, fragile. The occupation, in Britain, still lacks certain characteristics typical of the so-called higher professions, such as universal graduate entry. As a profession, it remains relatively powerless and poorly rewarded. This alone would count as evidence against my kind of interpretation of the Code. Yet this approach does encourage the recognition of the strategic importance that codes of conduct have in the process of professionalisation itself, and hence of the political context within which a code is interpreted.

The professional life world will incorporate assumptions about the actual and potential power of the profession. This may be explicated in terms of the idealism that is inherent in certain codes, and explicitly stated by the UKCC. The advisory documents published by the UKCC describe its *Code of Professional Conduct* as 'a portrait of the practitioner the Council believes to be needed and wishes to see within the profession'.[28] Yet this itself suggests something of the conservativism of the professional life world that grounds the Code. Implicit in the above statement is the expectation that nursing will develop principally through the excellence of its individual practitioners. The UKCC's Code contains little that relates to the resourcing of nursing. Paragraph ten in the second edition notes that the practitioner should have 'regard to the environment of care and its physical, psychological and social effects on patients/clients, and also to the adequacy of resources'. Within the context of trade unionism's assumptions, this paragraph might have been interpreted as a call for political action, including industrial action, in order to secure resources. It has since been changed.[29]

The social work codes are clear in their recognition of the problems of resourcing, and hence the profession's relationship to government. The BASW's code acknowledges the social worker's 'right and duty to bring to the attention of those in power, and of the general public, ways in which the activities of government, society or agencies create or contribute to hardship and suffering' (paragraph 9). NASW's code contains a broadly similar demand that the practitioner should be involved in public debate. Paragraphs VI.P.6 and 7 read: 'The social worker should advocate changes in policy and legislation to improve social conditions and to promote social justice. The social worker should encourage informed participation by the public in shaping social policies and institutions.'

CONCLUSION

I have argued that the interpretation of a code of conduct depends upon certain presuppositions current within the profession, and indeed outside of it. The precise formulation and wording of a code is of significance. There are extreme cases (as noted with a police force) in which the professional life world will lead to the 'ironisation' of the code, such that its tenets become meaningless. Yet even in these cases, the existence of the code, and its non-ironic interpretation by those outside the profession, are important. Such non-ironic interpretation, on the one hand, works to legitimate the legal monopoly of the profession, but on the other hand may be used to make professionals accountable to external, and more exacting, standards of morality. A code is a participant in any process of interpretation. If the members of the profession take the code literally, which may be regarded as typical in the 'caring' professions, then precise wording may encourage certain responses and forestall others. The British and American social work codes, on numerous points, provide models for such formulations.

In the case of the UKCC, the Code bears too many of the hallmarks of codes typical of conservative professions. The lack of adequate annotation, and too ready undermining of the pre-professional competences of its practitioners, including political competences, mean that the Council's interpretation of the Code must go largely unchallenged. The Code works merely to reinforce that which is already accepted, or that the Council wishes to see accepted, in the professional life world. The Code, it seems, is there to be taken for granted. This may tend to the unchallenged repro-duction of the hierarchy within the profession, for good or ill, and insulate the profession from an important critical resource, thereby paradoxically hindering the process of professionalisation.

While the sincerity of the Code is not to be doubted, the rigour with which it examines the professional life world, and more import-antly the degree to which it makes possible the problematising and consequent revision of that life world is questionable. It may be suggested that a profession that is denied its true status and re-sources should have a code that welcomes open debate and engagement, internally and externally.

NOTES

1 The other codes I refer to are those of the (American) National Society of Professional Engineers (NSPE), American Medical Association (AMA) and the Royal Pharmaceutical Society of Great Britain (RPS), and those of the British Association of Social Workers (BASW) and the (American) National Association of Social Workers (NASW), and the 1953 and 1973 codes of the International Council of Nurses (ICN). While this selection is in no way intended to be a representative sample of codes, it allows an initial comparison to be made between so-called higher and lower professions, between medical and non-medical profes-sions, as well as some international comparison. For the present, the difference between 'codes of ethics' or 'codes of conduct' will be overlooked.

2 United Kingdom Central Council for Nursing, Midwifery and Health Visiting, *The Code of Professional Conduct for the Nurse, Midwife and Health Visitor*, London: UKCC, 2nd edn 1984, 3rd edn 1992; UKCC, *Administration of Medicines*, London: UKCC, 1986; UKCC, *Confidentiality*, London: UKCC, 1987; UKCC, *Exercising Accountability*, London: UKCC, 1989; UKCC, '. . . with a view to removal from the register . . .', London: UKCC, 1990.

3 Downie, R. S. and Calman, K. C., *Healthy Respect: Ethics in Health Care*, London: Faber & Faber, 1987, p. 243.

4 Harris, J., *The Value of Life: An Introduction to Medical Ethics*, London: Routledge & Kegan Paul, 1985, p. 203.

5 Wieder, D. L., 'Telling the code', in R. Turner (ed.), *Ethnomethodology*, Harmondsworth: Penguin, 1974, pp. 161–2.
6 Habermas, J., *The Theory of Communicative Action*, vol. 2, *The Critique of Functionalist Reason*, Cambridge: Polity, 1987, pp. 113–98.
7 Schutz, A. and Luckmann, T., *The Structure of the Lifeworld*, London: Heinemann, 1974, p. 4.
8 The UKCC's document, *Exercising Accountability*, is meant to be a 'response' to requests received by the Council for an 'elaboration' of some of the clauses in the second edition of the Code. It raises further problems of interpretation.
9 Glazer, M., 'Ten Whistleblowers and How They Fared', *Hastings Center Report*, 1983, vol. 13 (6), pp. 33–41; and in Callahan J. C. (ed.), *Ethical Issues in Professional Life*, New York and Oxford: Oxford University Press, 1988.
10 Heywood Jones, I., *The Nurse's Code*, London: Nursing Times and Macmillan, 1990, p. 46.
11 See Muyskens, J. L., 'The Nurse as an Employee', in J. C. Callahan., op. cit. p. 310, and Muyskens, J. L., *Moral Problems in Nursing: A Philosophical Investigation*, Totowa, New Jersey: Rowman & Littlefield, 1982, pp. 168–78.
12 UKCC, '...with a view to removal from the register...', London: UKCC, p. 14.
13 See Jones, op. cit., pp. 18 and 20.
14 The 'Preamble' of the NASW code contains important qualifications of its presentation as a disciplinary tool. The demand is made that the 'code should not be used as an instrument to deprive any social worker of the opportunity or freedom to practise with complete professional integrity; nor should any disciplinary action be taken on the basis of this code without maximum provision for safeguarding the rights of the social worker'. The NASW code can be found as Appendix 1 of Minahan, A. *et al.*, *The Encyclopedia of Social Work*, Silver Spring, Md: National Association of Social Workers, 18th edn, 1987.
15 See Johnson, T. J., *Professions and Power*, London: Macmillan, 1972.
16 Kultgen, J., 'The Ideological Use of Professional Codes', in J. C. Callahan, op. cit., pp. 411–21; also in *Business and Professional Ethics Journal*, 1982, vol. 1 (3), pp. 53–69.
17 McKinlay, J., 'On the Professional Regulation of Change', in Halmos, P. (ed.), *Professionalisation and Social Change*, (Sociological Review Monograph No. 20), Keele: University of Keele Press, 1973, p. 308.
18 Similar phrases may be found in the codes of such disparate professions as social work – NASW speaks of 'appropriate channels' (V.M.2) – and engineering – NSPE speaks of 'employer or client and such other authority as may be appropriate', II.1.a.
19 UKCC, op. cit., 1989, p. 9.
20 Kultgen., op. cit., p. 415.
21 The fact that disciplinary hearings occur in public, as is the case with the UKCC's Professional Conduct Committee, must complicate this interpretation. It may be argued that public hearings serve only to publicise the competence of the profession in its self-regulation, albeit at some risk of intrusion by lay morality. However, the risk of intrusion is

significant and may be intentional and fruitful. The risk is exacerbated by the presence of lay members upon disciplinary or ethical committees.
22 See Downie and Calman, op. cit., pp. 57–8.
23 UKCC, op. cit., 1989, p. 16, my emphasis.
24 UKCC, op. cit., 1986, pp. 4, 7.
25 NASW, Code of Conduct, 1979, Preamble and VI.I.A.1.
26 UKCC, op. cit., 1989, p. 17. Since I wrote this the UKCC's Letter 24/1992 brings together, in two separate annexes, the revised editions of the Council's two key positions and policy statements on HIV/AIDS. Paragraph 22 of the Letter 'reminds those on its register that the first two clauses in its Code of Professional Conduct are a major part of the backcloth against which allegations of misconduct are judged and are not a formula for a practitioner to be selective about the categories of patient for whom he or she will care'.
27 UKCC, op. cit., 1989, p. 12.
28 UKCC, op. cit., 1987, p. 3.
29 Hunt has argued that the third edition's paragraph 11 has weakened such interpretations of the Code. See Hunt, G., 'Changing the Code', *Nursing Times*, 1992, vol. 88 (25), pp. 21–2.

Chapter 9

In the patient's best interests
Law and professional conduct

Ann P. Young

'I want to do something to help people' is a common response from student nurses when asked why they are entering nursing. Five years on, a proportion will already have left nursing and the remainder will have found that the context in which they are 'helping people' is not always conducive to the maintenance of high ideals.[1]

Although people always carry with them their own particular value systems and moral standards, nurse training socialises students to behave in a certain way and this also influences how nurses think and feel about what they are doing.[2] Sufficient dissonance with the individual's original attitudes and values may lead to the decision to leave nursing. Those who stay may have modified their expectations.[3]

This individual response occurs within the wider social context of both professional ethics and the law. 'Act always in such a manner as to promote and safeguard the interests and well-being of patients and clients' is the first and central statement of the nurse's *Code of Professional Conduct* and at first sight seems to embody what every nurse firmly believes in.[4] However, the law is a major influence on how nurses act and this chapter will explore how the law can seem to create potential conflict for the nurse in abiding by the Code.

I will first discuss at some length examples of how nurses behave in relation to the well-being of their patients, and then address this issue in relation to patients' interests.

THE INFLUENCE OF LAW

Both statute and case law have an influence on nurses' behaviour. The Nurses, Midwives and Health Visitors Act 1979 and 1992 set up the statutory framework in which nurses train, register and practice.

A few other examples of relevant statute law are the Abortion Act 1967, allowing for conscientious objection on the part of the nurse, the Mental Health Act 1983, giving nurses a special holding power in certain specified circumstances, and the Health and Safety at Work etc. Act 1974, requiring the employee to take reasonable care and to co-operate with others in maintaining health and safety.

The law also operates through a system of delegated legislation whereby certain named authorities are allowed to formulate statutory instruments, rules or orders which are then approved by the Secretary of State. For example, the Nurses' Rules 1983[5] and the Control of Substances Hazardous to Health (COSHH) Regulations 1986[6] have altered or extended the initial requirements of the Nurses, Midwives and Health Visitors Act 1979 and the Health and Safety at Work etc. Act 1974 respectively.

Case law

Of major importance to the nurse is case law. The law of tort (delict in Scotland) is part of the old unwritten common law and has been interpreted and clarified over the years through the court system. It is therefore often seen to be 'judge made', as the findings of judges in the higher courts become binding on later similar cases.[7] Two torts, negligence and trespass, have a major influence on nurses' behaviour and will be discussed at length later in this chapter.

As an example of the influence of case law, consider *R. v. Adams* 1957. Dr Adams was charged with the murder of an 81-year-old patient who had suffered a stroke. It was alleged that he had prescribed and administered such large quantities of heroin and morphine that he must have known that the drugs would kill her. The judge in the case stated,

> If the first purpose of medicine, the restoration of health, can no longer be achieved, there is still much for a doctor to do, and he is entitled to do all that is proper and necessary to relieve pain and suffering even if the measures he takes may incidentally shorten life.

Dr Adams was acquitted.[8] As a result of this, nurses need not fear prosecution if they follow the doctor's prescription of a potentially lethal dose of a drug as long as that amount of the drug is both necessary for and has been prescribed for the relief of suffering. Otherwise it would be more prudent to refuse to participate.

Modification of case law is dependent to some extent on the use of expert witnesses to inform the court of what is accepted professional practice in the particular circumstances of the case. This is one way in which judges can be informed of changes in practice so that the law can be amended.

Case law is also needed to interpret statute law. Statutes are usually drawn up to legislate over a broad range of circumstances and can never be worded in sufficient detail to answer every query that arises. For example, the Employment Protection (Consolidation) Act 1978 spells out in some detail the meaning of fair or unfair dismissal but still includes the words 'some other substantial reason of a kind such as to justify the dismissal' (S.57 (l)b). Cases have had to be brought to court to test the meaning of this phrase, often to the detriment of the employee.[9]

The need for additional regulatory mechanisms

A criticism of the law is that it is slow to respond to social changes. Although bills can be pushed through Parliament quickly where they have Government support, this is not the usual pattern of legislative change. Even Government bills are likely to be published initially as Green or White Papers for public consultation; for example, 'Working for Patients' (1989) led to the NHS and Community Care Act 1990.[10] Those issues not promoted by the Government will have to gain the support of a Member of Parliament who may put forward a Private Member's Bill of his choice. Even if successful at this stage, the pressure on Parliamentary time makes the chance of it reaching the statute books limited.

As already discussed, case law can be modified by the decisions of judges in the higher courts and respond to changes in professional practice through the use of expert witnesses. However, this is dependent on cases of relevance to nursing practice actually getting to court (many are settled out of court) so the process may be haphazard.

For these reasons there is often a need for additional or more detailed regulation of nursing practice. As shown, delegated legislation can be a means of providing this but is still fairly limited in practice and cannot be used to clarify the common law.

It is therefore not surprising that nurses find themselves turning to other mechanisms, both in the professional and employment arena, to guide their behaviour. The most responsive of these mechanisms to local need are the specific policies developed by each workplace, for example policies concerning drugs, complaints, discipline, sickness and uniforms. These are usually developed through a process of consultation between management and workers, represented by their unions. Their content must be within and may help to interpret the law, for example, a complaints policy will give the detail required by the Hospital Complaints Procedure Act 1985. Although they are not the law, failure to abide by a policy may have serious legal repercussions, including dismissal, as there is usually a stated contractual requirement to abide by them.

A number of statutes have additional guidelines drawn up to assist in their interpretation. Codes of practice are in existence to help interpret the various employment statutes, for example, relating to trade union activities. Although these are not the law, failure to abide by them could be criticised in an Industrial Tribunal and be detrimental to good employer/employee relations. Under Section 118 of the Mental Health Act 1983, 'the Secretary of State shall prepare and from time to time revise, a code of practice for the guidance of' doctors, managers and other professionals. The most recent Code of Practice of this kind was published in 1990.[11]

Of central importance to nurses is their *Code of Professional Conduct*, produced by the United Kingdom Central Council (UKCC) in response to its legal requirement 'to determine circumstances in which the means by which a person may, for misconduct ... be removed from the Register' (S.12 Nurses, Midwives and Health Visitors Act 1979). This code is 'issued to all registered nurses, midwives and health visitors' by the Council, 'which requires members of the professions to practise and conduct themselves within the standards and framework provided by the Code'.[12] Although not a legal document, a failure to abide by the Code can result in a hearing before the Professional Conduct Committee and removal or suspension from the Register, most assuredly a legal outcome.

Because of the non-legal nature of these additional regulatory mechanisms, there has to be a query as to how effectively they are implemented and enforced. An observer at an Industrial Tribunal will hear an employer criticised but not fined or otherwise penalised for breaching a relevant code of practice. Although the Mental Health Act Commission and the UKCC act as watchdogs, they can only respond to complaints brought to them. Local policies will only be seen as being forceful if linked with disciplinary action and possible termination of employment.

It has been suggested that one way of reinforcing the importance of the *Code of Professional Conduct* is to link this with the individual's contract of employment and some employers are doing just that. However, other employers are not yet ready to face the implications of raising the status of the Code in this way.

Negligence and standards of care

As already mentioned, the tort of negligence has a major influence on nurses' practice. For negligence, there must be a duty of care, a failure in that duty and resultant harm.[13] A key issue is the definition of what standard of care the law requires. 'The medical standard of care is the standard of a reasonably skilled and experienced doctor' (*Bolam* v. *Friern H. M. C.* 1957), and this concept of reasonableness applies to any professional in any situation.

In exploring the effect of negligence on nurses, a number of nursing decisions are influenced by a wish to avoid possible litigation. Harm can occur for a number of reasons, including the natural progression of a disease or an accepted risk of treatment, and on the whole the only issue here for the nurse is in ensuring that the patient is adequately informed. However, harm as a result of accidents causes great anxiety amongst professionals as it is here that the issue of negligence may take some teasing out. For example, if a patient falls out of bed and breaks an arm, is there negligence or not? The answer has to relate back to the reasonableness of the standard of care at the time. Close observation and precautionary measures would be expected if the patient was acutely ill and delirious, but not if the patient had previously been mentally alert and physically stable. This underlines the importance of sufficiently detailed nursing records to demonstrate that the care given by nurses was appropriate.

Any unusual circumstances must be recorded as these may have an effect on the standard of care that could be expected in the particular situation.

Conflicts may arise where nurses feel that resources are so inadequate that it is difficult to maintain a reasonable standard of care. Under the *Code of Professional Conduct*, the nurse must 'report to an appropriate person or authority any circumstances in which safe and appropriate care for patients and clients cannot be provided'.[14] There is a fear that complaining about insufficient staff or excessively heavy workloads could lead to victimisation (namely the Graham Pink case)[15] yet a failure to report such inadequacies can lead to criticism from the Professional Conduct Committee and a potential claim for negligence against either the nurses involved or the Health Authority. The case of *Bull* v. *Devon HA* 1989 is a useful example here.[16]

Delegation

Nurses are often under pressure to take on tasks or responsibilities that are new to them. There are two issues here. One relates to the acceptance of delegated functions, the other to the suitability or otherwise of the new tasks.

There is both a management and professional responsibility in the delegation of work. As the *Code of Professional Conduct* states, the nurse should 'acknowledge any limitations in your knowledge and competence and decline any duties or responsibilities unless able to perform them in a safe and skilled manner'.[17] The manager's responsibility is to check that she is not delegating inappropriately. The nurse can be negligent if harm results, the manager may also be negligent in delegation.

A problem may exist in recognising one's limitations. The inexperienced may not realise some of the potentially serious implications of performing certain functions inadequately. However, the law is absolutely clear on the responsibilities of those concerned. The Wilsher Case (*Wilsher* v. *Essex AHA* 1986–8) highlighted the point that inexperience can never be an excuse. The duty of care required by law is that expected of the post, not the postholder.[18] It therefore behoves a nurse inexperienced in a particular type of care to check her competence carefully, and if necessary, ask for training. The manager must also check, depending on the circumstances, either by asking for confirmation from the nurse as to her abilities or actually observing her perform the delegated functions competently.[19]

The nature of the tasks being delegated may also be of concern. The nurse has no right to refuse to accept delegated nursing tasks after the appropriate training has been offered (except in relation to abortion under the Abortion Act 1967). A refusal to give care on moral grounds can be overruled by the employer although it is hoped that with consideration and discussion a nurse could be supported in her beliefs. Certainly incidents have occurred, for example in refusing to participate in research, where non-co-operation on moral grounds has won the day.[20]

There is no doubt that the scope of professional practice is changing rapidly. Advances in research, alterations in the provision of health care and new approaches to professional practice all make demands on the nurse's skills. 'Practice must, therefore, be sensitive, relevant and responsive to the needs of individual patients and clients and have the capacity to adjust, when and where appropriate, to changing circumstances.'[21] This often involves the nurse undertaking a function normally performed by a doctor. The nurse may feel pressurised by both her medical and nursing colleagues to expand her role – after all, the more staff specifically trained for a function, the less the burden on individual members of staff. The Code itself states that the nurse should 'work in a collaborative and co-operative manner with health care professionals and others involved in providing care'.[22] The nurse will need to consider if it is in the patients' interest to adapt her role in the way suggested. Good standards of nursing care may become squeezed if additional resources are not made available.

Risk management

A final issue relating to patient safety concerns risk management in a situation of conflicting choices. It may be difficult to reach a conclusion as to what is overall in the patient's interests where each choice has both potential harm as well as potential benefit.[23] For example, as a patient is recovering from a suicide attempt, at what point is a decision to encourage independence preferable to continuing close supervision in order to prevent further self-harm? Both the law and the *Code of Professional Conduct* seem to emphasise safety. At first sight, therefore, they seem to support the provision of a safe environment and possibly a custodial approach. However, the harm of such an approach can be clearly demonstrated with both physical and mental health examples. The nurse has a responsibility to maintain and improve her knowledge and where both this and accepted practice support the importance of encouraging independence there can be clear arguments for a variety of actions. The professional duty is to have thought through these decisions with a legal proviso that to record their conclusions is also likely to be helpful.

PROMOTING AND SAFEGUARDING PATIENTS' INTERESTS

A major question has to be, whose interests? An assumption is often made by both doctors and nurses that decisions relating to care are made in response to the needs and wishes of the patient. While hoping that this is usually true, it is an assumption that is worth questioning. The issue of resources has already been mentioned in relation to negligence, but may also influence who is offered what treatments in a time of financial constraints. Individual values may lead to a misinterpretation of patient's wishes. For example, there may be a failure to accept that an elderly person would be willing to undergo major surgery or that a patient could refuse life-saving treatment. Where research is being undertaken, the patient may be pressured to participate, and when it is a question of discontinuing treatment, medical staff may be unduly influenced by the patient's relatives.

Consent

Much of the legal framework of patients' interests can be encompassed by the tort of trespass to the person, i.e. assault and battery (in their civil law meaning). A major legal defence against an action for trespass is consent and an important concept here is 'capacity'. 'The capacity to give a legally effective consent depends on the capacity to understand and come to a decision on what is involved, and the capacity to communicate that decision.'[24] How fully this conception is realised is debatable. (See Taplin's study in this volume.)[25]

Gaining consent is often seen as the business of doctors rather than nurses. For a number of reasons, this can be disputed. The significance of the nurse's professional responsibility in relation to patients' interests is underpinned by that first statement of the *Code of Professional Conduct*. Even legally, the nurse can and should have a role to play in the gaining of consent.

Consent can be implied, oral or written. In the giving of nursing care, consent is usually oral or assumed. The perception of most nurses is that they gain oral consent, for example in bathing, administering drugs, mobilising. Legally, the voluntary admission of a patient to hospital implies consent, and some subsequent actions of patients may also support this notion. It is possible that although nurses decry ever making the assumption that consent has been given, they may in fact make this assumption. A small-scale study showed that 'promoting individualised care is not necessarily synonymous with active patient involvement'.[26] The balance of power between nurse and patient may militate against true patient choice.

Medical care more often involves the gaining of written consent and is important where marked risks exist, for example general anaesthesia, surgery and some investigations. Nurses may find themselves assisting in this process. As already stated, consent involves understanding and coming to a decision on what is involved. The issue is very often one of sharing information and the nurse needs to understand the relevant legal framework.

A number of court cases have clarified the law in this area. A key case was *Bolam* v. *Friern H. M. C.* 1957. Mr Bolam was treated for his depression with electro-convulsive therapy (ECT) and suffered fractures in the course of this treatment. He alleged negligence in the failure to warn him of the risk. The judge found that the amount of information given accorded with 'accepted medical practice'. There would only have been negligence if Mr Bolam could have proved that further information would have led to him refusing consent.[27]

In a more recent case, *Sidaway* v. *Board of Governors of Bethlem Royal Hospital* 1984, similar conclusions were reached. Mrs Sidaway was not told that an operation to relieve neck pain was elective nor that it carried a 1 to 2 per cent risk of damage to the spinal cord. She was severely disabled and sued for battery. The claim was dismissed on the grounds that she had been told as much in 1974 as would have been accepted as proper by a body of skilled and experienced neurosurgeons. The doctrine of informed consent was rejected as being 'no part of English Law'.[28]

Consent and nurse advocacy

So what role can the nurse play? Although the nurse is unlikely to become involved in an action for battery, it is clear that she could be negligent if harm resulted from the giving of wrong information. Even so, there seem to be four possible actions available.

First, the nurse can clarify information already given. The patient is often in an extremely anxious state when the doctor is giving information and may misinterpret or not hear what has been said.

Second, additional information of a non-medical nature may assist the patient to reach a decision, for example, in relation to relevant nursing care or drug therapy.

Third, the nurse could give additional medical information but only if she is sure of the facts and experienced in that area of work. The potential difficulty here is that this may be contrary to the doctor's wishes and, as shown in the relevant case law, the doctor is very much in control of the medical information given. The nurse may face discipline for going against the doctor and the risk of this must be accepted if the nurse feels strongly that the patient has the right to certain facts.

Fourth, the nurse is to act as the patient's advocate. Advocacy means 'pleading the cause of another', and is possible within the legal framework of consent.[29] There is a responsibility on the doctor to answer questions put by the patient (*Sidaway* v. *Board of Governors of Bethlem Royal Hospital* 1984). Helping the patient to formulate and then ask appropriate questions of the doctor is an effective form of nurse advocacy. Being with the patient when the doctor is giving information is supportive and may enable the patient to feel more confident in questioning as well as enabling the nurse to enlarge on what is being said. The consent form suggested by the NHS Management Executive states that the patient may ask for a relative, friend or a nurse to be present.[30]

Patient advocacy schemes are still few and far between in England, but at least there is the beginning of awareness of their importance, particularly in the areas of obstetrics, paediatrics and mental health. Holmes writes, 'Advocacy is necessary because of an imbalance of power between the health service and its users. Members of the general public find it hard to criticise or question.'[31] The principle of 'citizen advocates' is seen as important for this reason, rather than the professional taking on this role.[32] As has already been pointed out in this chapter, the professional is subject to pressures and value judgements that may interfere with a clear interpretation of the patient's wishes. However, one may think it important that the nurse accepts this role in the absence of any better alternative and works hard to understand and counteract her own biases.

Patients unable to consent

There will always be a number of situations where the patient is unable to give consent to treatment or care. The patient who is unconscious is a clear example of this. However, nurses are frequently dealing with circumstances where there must be some debate over the capacity of the patient to give a valid consent or not and this difficulty may arise with children, the mentally ill and the mentally incapacitated.

The assessment of ability to give a valid consent appears to be left in the main to professional judgement and perhaps this is perfectly right and proper. However, the question has to be asked whose judgement and on what is this based? Nurses, by virtue of being with the patient for much longer periods of time than doctors, will be aware that a person's ability to understand may be variable over time and may also depend on the time taken both to communicate with the patient and to ascertain his understanding and wishes.

As was mentioned in relation to the fully competent patient, the professional's values may lead to undue influence on the patient, and this is likely to apply even more strongly where there is a possibility of some degree of incapacity. There may be a temptation to assume incapacity in order to override an unwanted patient response. As Culver and Gert suggest, 'a patient's apparently irrational refusal of consent should never be taken as a sign of incompetence if, were it to have been given in the same circumstances, the consent would have been regarded as valid'.[33] The legal framework in relation to a lack of capacity relies on several other defences against trespass to the person, and these have been developed particularly through case law.

In most cases, it is in the patient's interests to receive treatment or care that will save his or her life. The criteria of urgency and necessity can be used allowing doctors to carry out 'essential procedures which are necessary to save life or prevent serious damage to health'.[34] This does not mean to say that treatment has to be given.

In *Lim* v. *Camden and Islington AHA* 1979, a patient suffered a cardiac arrest after surgery. Although she was eventually revived, she suffered severe and irreversible brain damage. Lord Denning stated that after such an accident, those concerned were faced with an agonizing decision:

Is she to be kept live? Or is she to be allowed to die? Is the thread of life to be maintained to the utmost reach of science? Or should it be let fall and nature take its inevitable course? In such circumstances those about her should say – for mercy's sake, let the end come now.[35]

The 'urgency and necessity' defence is therefore not always a clear concept and there may well be times when professionals are not in agreement over its interpretation, particularly in relation to necessity. Although all concerned may claim to be working in the patient's interests, consensus may not be present, nor may even be sought by the doctors from other professionals involved in the patient's care. Indeed, there is no legal requirement to do so in these circumstances.

The ability of children to give consent has been debated in a number of venues. The Family Law Reform Act 1969 seemed to reinforce the importance of gaining consent from a parent or guardian for a child under the age of 16 years. However two pieces of law must put a different interpretation on this legislation. In *Gillick* v. *West Norfolk and Wisbech AHA and the DHSS* 1985, Lord Scarman stated that parental rights are derived from parental duties and these duties are only needed until the child is sufficiently capable of making his own decisions.[36] This seems to be a clear reflection on Skegg's definition of capacity to give consent, already stated. The Children Act 1989 replaces the concept of parental rights by one of parental responsibility and also attaches central importance to checking the 'ascertainable wishes and feelings of the child concerned where the child's welfare is under consideration'.[37]

Many misconceptions abound as to the rights of the mentally ill in relation to consent. Legally there is a difference depending on whether the patient has been admitted informally or detained under a Section of the Mental Health Act 1983. Informal patients are in the same position as any physically ill patient and even the detained patient can only be given treatment without his consent when it is urgent.[38] The nurse's responsibility in safeguarding these rights is extremely important. A number of sanctions can be brought to bear on the patient to encourage conformity to the nurse's or doctor's wishes. Failure of an informal patient to co-operate with treatment can be grounds for either discharging the patient from hospital or of invoking section five of the Act so that urgent treatment can then be given.

The third group of patients who are particularly vulnerable in the area of consent are those suffering from some organic brain dysfunction. Those with severe learning difficulties or with a disease such as Alzheimer's, may suffer from a long-term incapacity to give a valid consent.[39] It is therefore of only very limited use to invoke the defence of urgency and necessity and, where the patient is over 18 years, no other adult can give consent on his behalf. Decisions to treat very often had to be made without any legal guidelines.

The situation has now been clarified by several court cases involving the mentally handicapped. In *T*. v. *T*. 1988 the court supported the recommendations of the doctors that the woman have an abortion and be sterilised. In *F*. v. *West Berkshire HA* 1989, the judge declared that, as the mentally handicapped woman was unable to give consent because of her lack of capacity, a sterilisation operation could go ahead as it was in F's 'best interests'.[40]

There is now, therefore, in English law the notion of best interests of the patient where there is a long-term lack of capacity. In *Re F*, it was stated to be highly desirable as a matter of good practice to involve the courts in the decision to operate. Obviously it would be impossible and unnecessary to go to court for all decisions where patients' best interests have to be the deciding factor. This does leave a question as to how such decisions are made in practice.

The NHS Management Executive (1990) gives some advice.

> In practice, a decision may involve others besides the doctor. It must surely be good practice to consult relatives and others who are concerned with the care of the patient. Sometimes, of course, consultation with a specialist or specialists will be required; and in others, especially where the decision involves more than a purely medical decision, an inter-disciplinary team will in practice participate in the decision.[41]

Such practice would accord well with the nurse's *Code of Professional Conduct*. Unfortunately, as this document is only guidance, it does not give the nurse any authority to require her involvement. Legally, the courts have always supported the right of the medical profession to know what is best for their patients.[42]

Rights versus duties

One theme of this chapter has been the potential conflicts faced by the nurse in abiding by the *Code of Professional Conduct*. It seems that these conflicts operate on a number of levels.

At the legal level, there is a dilemma in following the law on negligence and that relating to battery. Negligence with its basis in duty of care emphasises the need to act in order to safeguard well-being. The right of the patient to say 'no', even if that decision leads to death, is not easy for the professional to accept but is supported by the law on trespass to the person. Balancing these rights and duties is often difficult. Will a failure to act be construed as negligence? Will a decision to overrule the patient's wishes be interpreted as an imposition on human rights?

The argument that if professionals act in the best interests of their patients this will provide protection against legal action, is attractive. As pointed out, such decisions are unlikely to be infallible and the nurse may have little voice in them.

At an employment level, further conflicts can arise. Not rocking the boat is seen in a time of high unemployment as increasingly important in order to keep one's job. Contractual obligations should mirror professional standards, and to some extent do. However, limited resources tend to lead to a standard that is fairly minimal in professional terms though usually acceptable legally. The requirement of audit in the National Health Service is a potential tool for exploring measures of quality.

The issue of accountability is also contentious. The nurse has accountability to her employer, the UKCC, the public, her patients and surely also to herself. As demonstrated repeatedly in this chapter, such multiple responsibilities will not be easy to balance. Accountability to self brings this chapter back to its starting point, the individual's own value systems and moral standards.[43]

A second important consideration in this chapter has been the question as to how effectively non-legal regulatory mechanisms can be implemented and enforced.

It is worth quoting in its entirety the UKCC's comment on Clause 1 of the Code, that the nurse shall 'act always in such a manner as to promote and safeguard the interests and well-being of patients and clients'. It goes on:

> It is recognised that, in many situations in which practitioners practice, there may be a tension between the maintenance of

standards and the availability or use of resources. It is essential, however, that the profession, both through its regulatory body (the UKCC) and its individual practitioners, adheres to its desire to enhance standards and to achieve high standards rather than to simply accept minimum standards. Practitioners must seek remedies in those situations where factors in the environment obstruct the achievement of high standards: to start from a compromise position and silently to tolerate poor standards is to act in a manner contrary to the interests of patients or clients, and thus renege on personal professional accountability.[44]

CONCLUSION

The statement given above is a strong one. It is to be hoped that nurses can be or become both assertive and political in ensuring the acceptance of their Code. The reality must be that such a task is extremely difficult, is not always supported by the legal and social culture in which nursing operates and glosses over some irreconcilable differences inherent in the interpretation of the Code.

Perhaps the conclusion has to be reached that the *Code of Professional Conduct* sets an unattainable standard. The nursing profession should be proud that this is the case.

NOTES

1 Dean, D. J., *Manpower Solutions*, London: Royal College of Nursing, 1987.
2 Cox, C., *Sociology, An Introduction for Nurses, Midwives and Health Visitors*, London: Butterworth, 1983.
3 Secord, P. and Backman, C., *Social Psychology*, London: McGraw-Hill, 1964.
4 United Kingdom Central Council for Nursing, Midwifery and health Visiting, *Code of Professional Conduct*, London: UKCC, 1992.
5 Statutory Instruments, Nurses, Midwives and Health Visitors, Rules Approval Order No. 873, 1983.
6 Health and Safety Commission, *Control of Substances Hazardous to Health Regulations*, London: HMSO, 1989.
7 Padfield, C., *Law made Simple* (revised by Smith, F. E.), 6th edn, London: Heinemann, 1983.
8 Cited in Skegg, P. D. G., *Law, Ethics and Medicine*, Oxford: Oxford University Press, 1984, p. 135.
9 Bercusson, B., *The Employment Protection (Consolidation) Act 1978*, London: Sweet & Maxwell, 1979.

10 Department of Health, *Working for Patients*, London: Department of Health, 1989.
11 DHSS, *Code of Practice, Mental Health Act 1983*, London: DHSS, 1990.
12 UKCC, op. cit., 1992, 'Notice' on last page. See Andrew Edgar's general critique of professional codes in his chapter in this volume.
13 See Padfield, op. cit.
14 UKCC, op. cit., 1992, sec. 12.
15 Turner, T., 'Crushed by the System', *Nursing Times*, 1990, vol. 86 (49), p. 19.
16 Tingle, J. H., 'The Important Case of Bull', *Nursing Standard*, 1990, vol. 4 (37), pp. 54–5.
17 UKCC, op. cit., 1992, sec. 4.
18 Tingle, J. H., 'Negligence and Wilsher', *Solicitors' Journal*, 1988, vol. 132 (25), pp. 910–11.
19 Young, A. P., *Law and Professional Conduct in Nursing*, London: Scutari, 1991, p. 56.
20 Tingle, J. H., 'Medical Paternalism: Blowing the Whistle', *Solicitors' Journal*, 1989, vol. 133 (44), p. 3.
21 UKCC, *The Scope of Professional Practice*, London: UKCC, 1992. See also Hunt, G. and Wainwright (eds), *Expanding the Role of the Nurse*, Oxford: Blackwell Scientific, 1994.
22 UKCC, op. cit., 1992, sec. 6.
23 Carson, D. and Montgomery, J., *Nursing and the Law*, London: Macmillan, 1989.
24 Skegg, op. cit., p. 48.
25 See also the earlier study: Byrne, D. J., Napier, A. and Cuschieri, A., 'How Informed is Signed Consent?', *British Medical Journal*, 1988, vol. 296, pp. 839–40.
26 Waterworth, S. and Luker, K. A., 'Reluctant Collaborations: Do Patients Want to be Involved in Decisions Concerning Care?' *Journal of Advanced Nursing*, 1990, vol. 15, pp. 971–6.
27 Brazier, M., *Medicine, Patients and the Law*, Harmondsworth: Penguin Books, 1987.
28 Faulder, C., *Whose Body Is It*? London: Virago, 1985.
29 *Chambers English Dictionary*, Cambridge: Chambers, 7th edn, 1988.
30 NHS Management Executive, *A Guide to Consent for Examination or Treatment*, London: Department of Health, 1990.
31 Holmes, P., 'The Patient's Friend', *Nursing Times*, 1991, vol. 87 (19), pp. 16–17.
32 Booth, W., 'A Cry for Help in the Wilderness', *The Health Service Journal*, 14 February 1991, vol. 101, pp. 26–7.
33 Culver, C. M. and Gert, B., *Philosophy in Medicine*, Oxford: Oxford University Press, 1982, p. 62.
34 National Consumer Council, *Patients' Rights: A Guide for N.H.S. Patients and Doctors*, London: NCC, 1983.
35 Cited in Skegg, op. cit., p. 151.
36 Brazier, op. cit., p. 226.
37 Leenders, F., 'Children First', *Community Outlook*, July 1990, pp. 4–6.

38 Young, A. P., *Legal Problems in Nursing Practice*, London: Chapman & Hall, 2nd edn, 1989.
39 Greengross, S. (ed.), *The Law and Vulnerable Elderly People*, Age Concern, London: Mitcham, 1986. See Maddie Blackburn's chapter in this volume.
40 Dimond, B., *Legal Aspects of Nursing*, London: Prentice Hall, 1990.
41 NHS Management Executive, op. cit., p. 10.
42 Young, op. cit., 1991, p. 25.
43 See Geoffrey Hunt's chapter on accountability in this volume.
44 UKCC, *Exercising Accountability*, London: UKCC, 1989, p. 7. For the relative merits and demerits of the third edition of the Code, which appeared in 1992, see the articles by Reg Pyne and Geoffrey Hunt in *Nursing Times*, 1992, vol. 88 (25), pp. 20–2.

Chapter 10

Nursing and the concept of care

An appraisal of Noddings' theory

Linda Hanford

INTRODUCTION

AIDS and the professional response to the pandemic have raised fundamental questions about the necessity for and the nature of lay and professional caring. The assertion made by some health care professionals that they should have the right to refuse to care for persons with HIV disease has raised questions about the nature of professional obligation and the meaning of care. Further, HIV disease has a large impact on women as care-givers, due to the pervasive cultural assumption that women have a natural aptitude for caring and that they will willingly assume such care.

In any case, 'care' is often said to be the central concept of nursing and it has received much attention from nursing theorists. Nel Noddings, an American educator and philosopher, is one of the theorists most frequently cited in scholarly work on caring done by other disciplines, although until the last few years her work had not been discussed in the nursing literature.[1] Using a 'feminine-feminist' approach, Noddings explores the question 'What does it mean to care and be cared for?' She argues that human caring and the memory of being cared for are the foundation of ethical response. Sara Fry, an American nurse philosopher, has stated that Noddings' work provides 'a viable theoretical framework that realistically represents the nature of the nurse–patient relationship'.[2] However, little work has been done to explore how Noddings' thesis might be applied to nursing.

In what follows I will give an exegesis of Noddings' theory, and offer some preliminary observations on how her work may be related to nursing in general, and to caring for persons with HIV disease in particular. One particular aspect of Nodding's theory, that of caring for strangers, or for those for whom one does not naturally care, will be explored in greater depth, in the context of our obligation to care for those with HIV disease. I will then give a critique of Nodding's theory and examine the relevance of an ethic of care for nursing.

CARING: A FEMININE APPROACH TO ETHICS

Following the work of Gilligan[3] on the differential moral reactions of men and women, Noddings develops her theory of caring from a feminine response; one rooted in the idea of human relationship. The approach to ethics through law and principle is seen as a masculine approach. Noddings describes the difference between masculine and feminine approaches to ethical concerns thus:

> Women, in particular, seem to approach moral problems by placing themselves as nearly as possible in concrete situations and assuming personal responsibility for the choices to be made. They define themselves in terms of caring and work their way through moral problems from positions of one-caring. . . . Further, the process of moral decision making that is founded on caring requires a process of concretisation rather than one of abstraction. An ethic built on caring is, I think, characteristically and essentially feminine – which is not to say, of course, that it cannot be shared by men, any more than we should care to say that traditional moral systems cannot be embraced by women. But an ethic of caring arises, I believe, out of our experience as women, just as the traditional logical approach to ethical problems arises more obviously from masculine experience.[4]

The focus is on ethical caring – how we meet each other morally. Ethical caring arises out of natural caring, from natural inclination or love. Natural caring is a relation perceived as good. This 'longing for goodness' motivates us to care in order to remain in the caring relation. Relation is taken as 'ontologically basic . . . we recognize human encounter and affective response as a basic fact of human existence' and the caring relation is seen as ethically basic.[5] Relation is defined as a 'set of ordered pairs generated by some rule that describes the affect – or the subjective experience – of the members'.[6] It is important to note that Noddings begins with caring as experienced and learned within the nuclear family, and goes on to expand this experience to other relationships.

Noddings coins the terms 'one-caring' and 'cared-for' to connote the two agents in the relation. Several dictionary definitions of care are cited by Noddings: a burdened mental state (anxiety, fear or solicitude for another); regard for or inclination towards some one or thing; charged with the welfare or protection of some one or thing. Elements of all these senses of caring are located in the relationship between the one-caring and the cared-for:

> The commitment to act on behalf of the cared-for, a continued interest in his reality throughout the appropriate time span, and the continued renewal of commitment over this span of time are the essential elements of caring from the inner view.[7]

Caring is accessible to us all. It is rooted in our earliest memories and experiences of being cared for, as well as subsequent caring experiences. Caring is complex, intricate and subjective; a displacement of interest from one's own reality to the reality of the other, says Noddings.[8]

Three elements characterise the caring relationship, and it is in these elements that the attractiveness of the theory for nursing can be found. They are receptivity, relatedness and responsiveness.

Three elements of caring

Receptivity is the acceptance or confirmation of the cared-for by the one caring. Noddings uses the term 'engrossment' to describe the internal response of the one-caring to the cared-for. This need not be intense or pervasive but must be present in the one-caring. Caring means considering living things' natures and ways of life, needs and desires; trying to apprehend the reality of the other. This other-orientation is part of the nurse's stance in approaching a patient. It is a desire to know and to help the patient. One form it may take is in the assessment phase, when the relationship is being established. The focus on the patient is intense, and the nurse uses cues from many sources. It may also be seen as a posture of unconditional positive regard, wherein a trusting relationship is established as the nurse demonstrates acceptance and an effort to understand the patient's reality.

Noddings speaks of the other being a 'possibility' for the one-caring: 'To be touched, to have aroused in me something that will disturb my own ethical reality, I must see the other's reality as a possibility for my own.'[9] This in turn arouses the feeling that one must do something to help the other. This idea of possibility, which Noddings derives from Kierkegaard, is not clearly developed in her book. She seems to suggest that the other may inspire us to be better than we are when we strive to help, but she may also mean the idea, more simply put, that 'This could be me.'

Both senses may be helpful in thinking about caring for those with HIV disease. For the most part, those suffering from HIV disease may not initially, or may never be perceived by the nurse as a possibility for her reality, as in many cases either their sexual orientation and life-style, or their drug misuse may render them well outside her ken. Thus the articles in both the nursing and the lay press, which attempt to explain and put a human face on those suffering from HIV disease, are an effort to allay fear and promote understanding and tolerance. This will be discussed further in the section about caring for strangers or those who arouse negative feelings in the one-caring.

Relatedness is basic – the relation of the agents as a fact of human existence, in the case of nursing, as a *raison d'être* – without patients there would be no nurses. Noddings speaks of formal relationships which are in part rule-governed, in which the disposition to care is already present. The question becomes what does the fact of relationship entail about obligations? One answer to the question 'Why should I care for persons with HIV disease?' is 'Because you're a nurse.' The nurses' *Code of Professional Conduct* asserts that,

> You [the nurse] . . . must recognise and respect the uniqueness and dignity of each patient and client, and respond to their need for care, irrespective of their ethnic origin, religious beliefs, personal attributes, the nature of their health problem or any other factor.[10]

This statement begs ethical questions of role and duty. Noddings would assert that care is prior to either.

Responsiveness is the commitment of the one-caring to the cared-for. This involves a 'motivational shift' in the one-caring, a displacement away from self and towards the cared-for. The one-caring becomes available to the cared-for, is present to and focused on him. This displacement varies in conditions, time-span and intensity, as well as the nature or proximity of the one-caring to the cared-for. In this lies the richness of the theory in describing the nature of nursing and the nurse–patient relationship.

One condition affecting the level of commitment of the one-caring may be the degree of need of the patient for nursing care. People with HIV disease fluctuate in their demand for care due to the nature of the trajectory of HIV infection. Care may not be needed for long periods of good health after sero-conversion, but needed acutely around the testing phase, and periodically during exacerbation of the many expressions of the syndrome. Care at home has proved to be much more common than hospitalisation. The kind of relationship established during an acute, brief encounter is different in style and content than that developed over chronic or repeated admissions. The commitment to the cared-for usually deepens and develops with time and intimacy. All caring situations entail risk; the one-caring may be overwhelmed or undergo a conflict of obligations. This raises questions about the appropriate level of professional involvement. The involvement of many health care professionals and specialists causes fragmentation of the caring relationship, and there is a need to establish a pattern of care which guarantees continuity over the trajectory of the illness.

Those caring over a long period of time for persons with HIV disease have to contend with repeated involvement, intimacy and bereavement, as well as an increased risk of occupational exposure and concern about obligation to family which this entails.

Noddings' theory offers a challenge for nursing administration to create environments where nurse and patient, as well as nurse and nurse, may meet one another as moral beings, to be fully present one to the other. The possibility of the survival of the ethic of caring in nursing depends in part upon such organisational matters as consistency of nurse–patient assignment and resultant continuity of care which affords the time and space to develop a caring relationship. Management must value the developing relationship, and encourage the practice of caring behaviours. This means the abolishing of task-oriented nursing and an approach to health care which promotes the practitioners' autonomy of thought and action. Primary nursing is one style of care delivery which can do this. Finally, the administrator and nurse must meet each other as moral beings in a non-coercive, supportive manner, as ones-caring and cared-for.

Caring and repugnance

Caring is not always natural. The caring one feels for one's child is unlikely to be the same as the care one feels for a friend, or for what

Noddings' calls the 'proximate stranger'. This raises questions of the limits to our obligation to care. There is a state of 'readiness to care' in formal relationships, such as in the nurse–patient relationship. The ethic of nursing has to be understood from the perspective of the nurse–patient relationship.

Nurses' ability to care for people with HIV disease is challenged by the fact that many (but certainly not all) of those who contract the virus have done so because they have engaged in actions that some find repugnant. Prejudices against homosexuality are deeply rooted. Reactions to those who misuse drugs are also strong. Yet it is a firmly-held tradition in nursing, enshrined in every code of professional conduct, that nurses provide care without prejudice to their patients, regardless of race, gender, creed or health problem. How, then, can nurses resolve the attitudes which they may have with their professional duties and obligations?

Noddings, in developing her theory of caring as the foundation of ethical response, differentiates between states of caring wherein we care 'naturally' and those when we must make an effort to care. She talks about receiving the other empathically as we understand his or her reality.

> But receiving the other as he feels and trying to do so are qualitatively different modes. In the first, I am already 'with' the other. My motivational energies are flowing toward him and, perhaps, toward his ends. In the second, I may dimly or dramatically perceive a reality that is a repugnant possibility for me. Dwelling in it may bring self-revulsion and disgust. Then I must withdraw. I do not 'care' for this person. I may hate him, but I need not. If I do something in his behalf – defend his legal rights or confirm a statement he makes – it is because I care for my own ethical self. In caring for my ethical self, I grapple with the question: Must I try to care? When, and for whom?[11]

Must I, as a nurse, try to care? When and for whom? Some might think it sad that these questions have to be entertained at all in nursing. This question does not reflect any new crisis in nursing; the difficulty of caring for someone for whom we do not naturally care has been part and parcel of nursing practice since its inception as a professional endeavour.

However, as is the case in many issues, HIV/AIDS has become the prism through which many long-standing problems in the health care system are being seen. Nursing practice entails caring for strangers. When people enter the profession, their motivation very often is a desire to help others. They stand ready to care. We respond to their suffering and are motivated to relieve it. But there are those who come to nurses for care for whom it may be difficult to care naturally. They may be dirty, impolite, abusive, uncooperative or ungrateful. Nurses may find their way of living repulsive; some patients may have even seriously harmed others by their actions. How do nurses respond to this, and how should they respond?

I think that in these situations many nurses withdraw. If they do not withdraw physically, that is, refuse to care for this patient at all, they most certainly withdraw their emotional involvement. We might say they do not really have their heart in it. They become less friendly, more reserved, perhaps remaining merely civil. But such a response is crucial in the caring process. I believe that a deficiency in caring works against the possibility of true healing. Diseases can be cured by the skilful application of technical and chemical means, but the illness, regarded as an affront to one's sense of self, requires that the patient be met with sympathy as a suffering individual and helped to find meaning in his experience, in order that it be accommodated or resolved.

Natural caring

Does it make sense to say that the rationale for remaining in relation with the person against whom we feel strongly is 'caring for my ethical self'? This concept of an ethical self is crucial to Noddings' theory.

Noddings differentiates between 'natural' caring and 'ethical' caring.

> The focus of our attention will be on how to meet the other morally. Ethical caring, the relation in which we do meet the other morally, will be described as arising out of natural caring – that relation in which we respond as one-caring out of love or natural inclination. The relation of natural caring will be identified as the human condition that we, consciously or unconsciously, perceive as 'good'. It is that condition toward which we long and strive, and it is our longing for caring – to be in that special relation – that provides the motivation to be moral. We want to be moral in order to remain in the caring relation and to enhance the ideal of ourselves as one-caring.[12]

The ethical self is an ideal picture of what I might be, 'an active relation between my actual self and my ideal self as one-caring and cared-for'.[13]

Noddings appears to be influenced by the view of the philosopher David Hume, that morality is rooted in sentiment or feeling. She says that caring is a feeling that is universal in humans as a result of being cared for as a child. There are two feelings: the initial, enabling sentiment of natural caring, and a second sentiment in response to the first, which is the motivating feeling of 'I must' in reaction to the plight of another, set against the conflicting desire to serve one's own interests. She thinks that natural caring, or love, has no moral content in itself, and agrees with Kant that the ethical is always done out of duty and not out of love.

One might take issue with Noddings. That everyone feels this caring sentiment is open to question. The ability to care appears to be a matter of degree in different people. Furthermore, not every child has had caring, nurturing parents. But reactions differ. Some might grow up to be very uncaring while in others the longing for care might issue in a need for caring relationships. There is a view that many of those who enter helping professions do so to meet some need which is lacking in themselves. Also, caring experiences may be derived from sources other than the mother–child relation.

Ethical caring

Noddings grounds her ethic of caring in the response to the feeling that I must do something to help another (even if I do not have the natural inclination). Ethical caring depends on natural caring in this way: if one were incapable of natural caring (as with the psychopath) then one could not be capable of ethical caring. But ethical caring is different from natural caring in that it is an acknowledgement that one ought to do something even if one does not want to, because one feels that one must choose to be one's 'best self', one must try to sustain a caring attitude in general. Ethical caring, then, requires the recognition of an ideal self and the commitment to realise that self.

Noddings argues that one is obliged to act on the 'I must' because of the value one places on the kind of relatedness involved in caring. 'The genuine moral sentiment . . . arises from an evaluation of the caring relation as good, as better than, superior to, other forms of relatedness.' This obligation is governed by two criteria:

the existence of or potential for present relation, and the dynamic potential for growth in relation, including the potential for increased reciprocity and, perhaps, mutuality. The first criterion establishes an absolute obligation and the second serves to put our obligations in an order of priority.[14]

The first criterion is met, I suppose, by the patients who happen to be in the nurse's care. Here, assuming the patient 'is capable of responding as cared-for' and that the nurse can receive this response, the obligation is quite unconditional. One might object that this is after all conditional on the capability of the nurse, or on the availability of the requisite time and skill. But the point is that if a particular nurse cannot herself meet a patient's need, then she must ensure that someone else does if possible. She sees its absoluteness.

The second criterion is met by people, for example sick children in the Third World, to whom I may feel some obligation, but which I am free to accept as an obligation depending on all sorts of factors. To respond to them fully, for example, I might have to give up nursing the patients I have, and even then I could only respond to some and not to all. I would have to prioritise.

'Reciprocity' creates some difficulties for nursing, I think, because it is not necessarily a feature of the nurse–patient relationship. Essentially this relationship is a meeting of unequals. The patient comes to the nurse for care, not vice versa. Caring takes place by the nurse without the expectation that the patient will in turn care for her or consider her personal development. Of course, this is not to deny that the cared-for may still respond, by growing under care, or by demonstrating any of the thousands of responses that lets the nurse know that her caring has been effective (quiet rest after pain relief, for example). But what of the patient who cannot, due to physiological or mental obstacles, respond to the nurse? Does that absolve her of the obligation to care? Surely not. In fact one might argue for an enhanced duty in view of the patient's vulnerability.

Ethical caring is summoned when natural caring fails. One must then try to care, according to Noddings, because one is in the relation with another. One might try to see the other's reality differently by looking at it 'objectively'. Admittedly, 'this sort of looking does not touch my own ethical reality; it may even distract me from it'.[15] To illustrate, in the case of the HIV patient for whom P happens to feel repugnance, P can try to care in a different fashion. P could learn more about homosexuality or drug abuse, view them in social and historical context. Some knowledge of the frequency of heterosexual anal intercourse may change P's view that it is abnormal or 'unnatural'; death rates and bereavement rates among gay communities may shock and bring compassion. In this way P may come to appreciate the stresses involved. The effort to understand, may lead to placing oneself in the other's shoes, may evoke caring.

Then again, it may not make P care. Intimate knowledge of homosexual behaviour and the drug culture may deepen the revulsion previously felt, or may harden attitudes to drug misusers. Again, Noddings would say that, in this case, one does not care and must withdraw. But a middle ground appears possible in Noddings' scheme, which I will now go on to discuss.

Diminished ethical capacity

Ethical behaviour is marked by feeling, thinking and acting as one-caring. It depends in part on the degree of receptivity the one-caring has effectively exercised. One may fail to receive the other accurately or adequately. One may be preoccupied, or hearing and seeing selectively. For whatever reason, one may not wish to be, or not be able to be, fully with the other. In this case, Noddings says, one is in a state of diminished ethical capacity.

One can care meaningfully for only so many people. Noddings is clear that the primary obligation and deepest caring generally occurs in the family, the inner circle of caring. The one-caring, for whatever reason, may have to 'retreat' to this circle, 'consciously excluding particular groups', either for self-preservation or 'to maintain the quality of the ideal for the remaining cared-fors'.[16] In nursing, one may find that in sustained giving over a period of time to patients who require intense involvement, one turns to friends and family for support and restoration of one's self. As nurse–patient relationships are not equal, in that the patient does not give to the nurse the caring she requires, the nurse may get her 'caring well' refilled in more equal relationships. This quantitative diminishment of caring can be most pragmatically demonstrated by the nursing staff shortage. Nurses are required to take care of more and more patients, and consequently they can give a diminishing amount to each. In a very real sense, nursing is practising in a chronically ethically diminished state.

Qualitative ethical diminishment, for Noddings, seems to entail some form of rejection of the impulse to care, or acting contrary to one's moral beliefs. Noddings uses the extreme example of a woman who has killed her husband in self-defence, feels guilty about it, and may be regarded as in a permanently ethically flawed state. Noddings addresses the question of when one is justified in withdrawing from caring, but the criteria she proposes seem me to be too stringent: 'She must meet the other as one-caring until he is, intentionally, a positive threat to her physical or ethical self. Then, and only then, she must withdraw.'[17] Even in withdrawing, the one-caring must preserve the possibility of future caring if she can, and must not interfere with his being cared for by others.

It is difficult to imagine a situation where a person with HIV disease would, intentionally, threaten a nurse's person or her ethical self, although it is not impossible. Certainly, nurses are not required to remain in a threatening situation, although they are often taught techniques (in psychiatric nursing, for example) to prevent or escape such threats. One does not usually get cytomegalovirus (CMV), a viral infection associated with AIDS, intentionally transmitted to one. Still, the presence of CMV in a patient is a legitimate reason for a pregnant nurse to withdraw her services. Further, there is a strong obligation to ensure that patients are not abandoned, which perhaps goes further than the mere non-interference proposed by Noddings.

The ethical ideal

The ideal which guides ethical caring is a picture of goodness: 'I see that when I am as I need the other to be toward me, I am the way I want to be – that is, I am closest to goodness when I accept and affirm the internal "I must".'[18] This picture of goodness is a personal construct of what I might be. Noddings writes:

> The ethical self is an active relation between my actual self and a vision of my ideal self as one-caring and as cared-for. It is born of the fundamental recognition of relatedness; that which connects me naturally to the other, reconnects me through the other to myself. . . . The characteristic 'I must' arises in connection with this other in me, this ideal self, and I respond to it. It is this caring that sustains me when caring for the other fails, and it is this caring that enables me to surpass my actual uncaring self in the direction of caring.[19]

As this personal construct is rooted in the experience of relationships, it follows that it is subject to growth and change (and, presumably, degeneration) based on the character of those relationships. This leads Noddings to suggest ways of nurturing and maintaining this ideal. Receptivity and relatedness are developed in one by talking about one's feelings and active listening to others. Dialogue is central. It appears that in this sense, the groundwork can be laid for effective caring by teaching and role-modelling, something that is a part of many nursing curricula.

Noddings speaks of the possibility of always attributing the best possible motives to the cared-for. This functions to raise the appraisal of the other, rather than to lower it. In this way the cared-for feels received and valued. It would seem also that the one-caring would feel good about life and herself in holding such a positive outlook. She also speaks of the possibility of a person maintaining the ideal by an attitude which celebrates rather than decries the ordinary in human living as 'the source of her ethicality and joy', her wonder and appreciation of living.

She further discusses the need for the moral agent to be 'in condition' to care, needing adequate rest and relaxation. Presumably the overworked and exhausted nurse is in no condition to be sensitive and caring.

CRITIQUE OF NODDINGS

Moral end

The major objection I have to Noddings' ethic of caring is that she often speaks as though morality serves some general purpose outside itself. Thus she gives an account of caring in terms of attaining certain ends. One of these is realising an ideal or picture I have of myself. Another is remaining 'in relation', fear of falling out of relation with others. Yet another is satisfying certain basic needs (feelings) that I have as a human being.

The question of whether there is a moral end, and if so, what it is, is a major theme in moral philosophy. The philosopher J. L. Stocks has argued that it is quite mistaken to think of morality in this way. Stocks says that any action done because the agent thinks it right to do so already has moral significance. Seeing the action as right does not, for Stocks, entail that there is some purpose or end to the act in question which gives it its value. Of course, in doing what I consider to be the right thing I may aim to achieve a certain end, but it is not the end itself which makes the action moral. Stocks points out rightly that 'purpose alone will never fully justify action to itself'.[20]

We must ask whether it really makes sense to talk about ethical caring (trying to care) as a means to the end of the development of one's ethical self. Caring may have this result, but it is surely not this result that makes the caring ethical. To give an account of caring as a moral attitude in terms of any purpose, whether it be to heal the other, or to develop the ethical self, would be, on Stocks' account, 'incomplete and defective'.[21] Why is this so?

First, 'the claims of morality, as they operate in human life, present on the face of it a very different appearance from the claims of policy or purpose'.[22] These claims often involve a duty to act, or refrain from acting, often requiring the constraint of one's desires or one's own purposes. Some acts are good in themselves, regardless of their purpose or end. One might say that caring is just good, and requires no justification.

Let us take as an example, the institutional and professional policy which requires that a patient should not be abandoned. Let us say a nurse feels that, despite the policy, she cannot care for a person suffering from HIV disease because it is repugnant to her. In Noddings' terms, she certainly does not care 'naturally' and, despite trying, cannot bring herself to care 'ethically', cannot attain the purpose of realising her 'best self'. But if we were to disapprove of this nurse's position surely that does not necessarily have anything to do with her failure to realise some purpose or policy. We may simply think she is prejudiced, insensitive, uncaring, or even callous and that is sufficient to make ourselves understood. Characterising her behaviour in this way is to point to a failure to keep certain purposes (desires, fears, etc.) in check. It is not another purpose that could keep them in check, it is moral considerations such as compassion or concern.

In this case, the nurse may meet the institutional policy by arranging for someone else to do the caring; she may even feel that this arrangement has ensured that her 'best self' has not been compromised. But that need make no difference to our justifiable disapproval of her, and our regarding her behaviour as a moral failure. To cite Stocks: 'Purpose will not yield "right" and "wrong".'[23]

Second, judgements of the effectiveness of actions are not the same as judgements of their moral value or disvalue. In the example, the nurse may act quite effectively, indeed it may be much more effective for someone else to care for the patient than for her to do so, but again that does not effect my moral failure – which resides in the fact that I have evaded my moral responsibility.

Third, motive plays a central role in the moral judgement of action. But, says Stocks, 'Purpose excludes motive from moral judgment.'[24] To return to the example. If we consider the motives of the nurse it seems reasonable to suspect that her motive is to avoid having to do what she considers 'a dirty job' or perhaps a 'risky' one. This is one reason, or the reason, why many would be morally disapproving of her behaviour. To look at it another way, we often excuse people for achieving or attempting to achieve misconceived purposes when we know that their motives were good. A nurse who sincerely thought that the best way to care for an HIV/AIDS patient was to avoid all medication and rely on prayer might be regarded as incompetent or stupid or even as a menace, but no one could claim that she was evil – her motives were good.

Stocks directly addresses the notion of 'self-affirmation or self-realisation' as a purpose or end or answer to the question 'Why should I be moral?' This question touches upon Noddings' conception of caring as aiming at one's 'best self'. Stocks views the notion as obscuring the essential nature of morality by emphasising development towards some future state which, he says, 'is irreconcilable with the data of the moral consciousness'.[25] One's moral perfection as an end is not the highest good, nor can it be the only good.

The feminine basis

Noddings can also be criticised for a misconception of the provenance of caring. One might consider whether it is a natural, essentially human (or female) feeling or sentiment, or whether it is a set of attitudes or behaviours which are learned or socially mediated. By claiming that it is a natural, innate sentiment, her work raises questions about universality and causes. In recent writings, she has backed off from the position that caring is a natural attribute and is now willing to accept that it may be experiential:

> We need not trace these differences [in moral stances between women and men] beyond experience to essential differences in nature. This leaves open the possibility of both reconciliation (through an appreciation of differing experience and commit-

ments) and transcendence (by uncovering what is shared beneath the surface conflicts).[26]

Noddings now sees the purpose of elucidating a theory of caring as not to claim moral superiority for women (this was a strong feature of her book), but to improve moral life by adding to it the feminine perspective.

Noddings has relied heavily on the work of Carol Gilligan in her view that women's moral judgements are rooted in a caring attitude, context and connection, and on the work of psychologist Carl Jung, who attributed the moral differences between men and women to essential, predetermined nature. Her insistence on the feminine nature of caring, and her valuing it as morally superior to the 'masculine justice-centred ethic' is attractive to those in some quarters of nursing who insist that caring is the distinguishing characteristic of nursing (doctors diagnose, treat and cure). This may be seen as an effort to establish nursing as a distinct discipline currently undergoing professionalisation. I do not think that this extreme kind of turf-cutting is either helpful or necessary.

Yet even Gilligan has since modified her position in the light of ongoing research that shows that care-based and justice-based attitudes are shared by men and women.[27] Her work had been seen by many feminists as a convincing argument for the existence of a distinct women's morality, despite Gilligan's assertion that the ethic of care is not a category of gender difference. It is now widely accepted that a justice-based or care-base orientation has more to do with the type of moral situation encountered by individuals, although it remains true that men and women may tend to focus on, or emphasise, different moral aspects of a situation.[28]

Attempts have been made to demonstrate empirically that moral attitudes are rooted in gender, and some of these might be thought to show that Noddings was right in the position taken in her book. But there are methodological problems. The studies have been too small, using small samples and different instruments for which psychometric properties have not been established. In other words, different studies, looking at related but different phenomena, using different methods yield different results, which are then used by competing scholars to challenge the validity of each other's findings.

Tronto, a political scientist, says that what is important is the adequacy of the ethic of care as a moral theory, and not gender difference. She warns of three drawbacks of positing a special link between 'care' and 'the feminine'.

1 This link is doubtful since the evidence to support gender-related moral difference is inadequate.
2 It is a politically dangerous position for women in that the assertion of a gender difference 'in a social context that identifies male as normal' implies the inferiority of the female.
3 It is 'philosophically stultifying' as one becomes trapped trying to defend women's morality rather than looking critically at the care (and, I would add, at actual nursing practice).[29]

An important alternative view of gender and moral development is that it has been structured by the social construction of generations of oppression. Whereas nursing's rise to professional status is inextricably linked to that of feminism, this view merits further exploration in light of nursing and medicine as a master/slave relationship, the oppression of gay people, and the marginalisation of others affected by HIV disease. For instance, the master/slave morality gives rise to an impoverished idea of care as mere service, uninformed by free judgement owing to a lack of choice about whom or what is to be served. This may lead nursing into self-deception, denying its impotence in relation to its professed values and aims.[30]

CONCLUSION

No doubt one has to be somewhat suspicious of theories of morality, all of which are reductionist in one way or another. One can understand that theories like Noddings' are attractive to nurses because they not only put 'care' and women's concerns at the centre, but they present morality as a coherent unitary domain and advance the simple idea that there is one type of ideal moral personality, a best way to reason morally. This oversimplified view is reminiscent of the idea that there is 'one best way' in nursing, that there ought to be a theory of nursing, one best curriculum, one best nursing research and so on. This is more comfortable than dealing with the pluralism, complexity, and rich diversity of moral life.

My general view is that Noddings' theory is too narrow and rigid a conception to encompass the moral situation of nursing. However, it does offer important initial insights into 'care' as a concept that is especially significant to nursing.

NOTES

1 Noddings, N., *Caring: A Feminine Approach to Ethics and Moral Education*, Berkeley and Los Angeles: University of California Press, 1984.
2 Fry, S. T., 'Toward a Theory of Nursing Ethics', *Advances in Nursing Science*, 1989, vol. 11 (4), p. 16.
3 See Gilligan, C., *In a Different Voice*, Cambridge, Mass.: Harvard University Press, 1982.
4 Noddings, p. 8.
5 ibid., p. 4.
6 ibid., pp. 3–4.
7 ibid., p. 16.
8 ibid., p. 14.
9 ibid.
10 United Kingdom Central Council, *Code of Professional Conduct*, London: UKCC, 1992, sec. 7.
11 Noddings, op. cit., pp. 17–18.
12 ibid., p. 5.
13 ibid., p. 49.
14 ibid., pp. 83, 86.
15 ibid., p. 14.
16 ibid., p. 115.
17 ibid., p.115.
18 ibid., p. 49.
19 ibid., pp. 49–50.
20 Stocks, J. L., *Morality & Purpose*, London: Routledge & Kegan Paul, 1969, p. 72.
21 ibid.
22 ibid., p. 73.
23 ibid.
24 ibid., p. 75.
25 ibid., p.77.
26 Noddings, N., 'Do we Really Want to Produce Good People?', *Journal of Moral Education*, 1987, vol. 16 (3), p. 181.
27 Card, C., 'Women's Voices and Ethical Ideals: Must we Mean What we Say?', *Ethics*, 1988, vol. 98, pp. 125–35.
28 See Omery, A., 'Moral Development: a Differential Evaluation of Dominant Models', *Advances in Nursing Science*, 1983, vol. 6 (1), pp. 1–17; Bebeau, M. J. and Brabeck, M. M., 'Integrating Care and Justice Issues in Professional Moral Education: A Gender Perspective', *Journal of Moral Education*, 1987, vol. 16 (3), pp. 189–203; Flanagan, O. and Jackson, K., 'Justice, Care and Gender: the Kohlberg–Gilligan Debate Revisited', *Ethics*, 1987, vol. 97, pp. 622–37; Okin, S. M., 'Reason and Feeling in Thinking About Justice', *Ethics*, 1989, vol. 99, pp. 229–49.
29 Tronto, J. C., 'Beyond Gender Difference to a Theory of Care', *Signs*, 1987, vol. 12 (4), pp. 644–63.
30 Card, op. cit., p. 130.

Chapter 11

'Medical judgement' and the right time to die

Anne Maclean

I shall examine, from a philosophical point of view, a pattern of argument which emerges from time to time in discussions of euthanasia. The argument may be described as an attempt to place euthanasia outside the bounds of medicine; euthanasia, it claims, does not fall within the remit of medical practice, of what doctors do as doctors. This is because it involves judgements and decisions which it is not the business of a doctor as a doctor to make. Doctors are in the business of making medical judgements and decisions and the decision to hasten a patient's death – to kill a patient – is not a medical decision but a moral decision. This is not the case with a decision to withhold treatment from a certain patient, or to withdraw treatment once it has begun. These are (or can be) medical decisions, decisions which doctors as doctors are entitled to make. 'We should stop treating this patient's cancer' or 'We should not attempt to cure this patient's pneumonia' – these can be legitimate medical judgements. 'We should give this patient a lethal injection' can never be a legitimate medical judgement, not because it happens always to be illegitimate but because it is not a *medical* judgement at all. It is a moral judgement. Doctors as doctors are not entitled to make judgements of this kind.

Health carers who are not doctors but, for example, nurses, may be inclined to think that a discussion of this argument can have little to do with their professional concerns; as we shall see, however, this is not the case.

TWO KINDS OF JUDGEMENT?

Central to the argument outlined above is a distinction between two distinct types or kinds of judgement and decision: medical, on the one hand, and moral (or, more generally, evaluative) on the other. The claim is that judgements of the latter type fall outside medicine and that such judgements as 'we ought to give this patient a lethal injection' are of this type. Thus although the withdrawal or with-holding of treatment may be medically indicated, euthanasia – hastening death – can never be medically indicated.

I shall argue that the distinction between medical judgements and moral judgements upon which this argument relies cannot be sustained.

Whose argument is the argument I have described? In exactly the form that I have stated it, I doubt if it is anyone's. Nevertheless it is not a figment of my imagination. I have encountered arguments along these lines in the writings of several people and also in conversations with health care professionals. I am going to structure my criticism of this argument around some passages from a well-known book written by a doctor, Richard Lamerton's *Care of the Dying*.[1]

Something like the argument I have sketched does appear in this book in connection with the idea of 'the right time to die' (which is the title of chapter 8). It may be that Dr Lamerton would disown the view that I am about to attribute to him, in which case I tender my apologies in advance. What matters, it seems to me, is that this view is held, and I think it is important to come to grips with it.

Dr Lamerton says of 'the right time to die':

> It is proposed that there is a right time to die, that this time may come before a man has breathed the very last breath of which his body is capable, and that an experienced physician can recognise or learn to recognise that the right time to die has come. Please understand that what is proposed is to refrain from prolonging life beyond the right time, *not* to hasten the termination of life in any way.[2]

Dr Lamerton is himself very much opposed to euthanasia. I am not going to take issue with his moral views; but I do have philosophical objections to the argument of the chapter referred to above. In the passage quoted, there is the suggestion that the right time to die is a matter of medical judgement only, the judgement of an 'experienced physician'. There are similar suggestions throughout the book. We read of 'good medicine', 'legitimate medical decisions', 'clinical judgement' as 'our only guide' and of 'appropriate and inappropriate treatment'. Of particular importance is the claim that: 'the withdrawal of artificial means of prolonging life . . . is not euthanasia, it is just good medicine. It is merely acting upon a recognition that a test, a trial of therapy, has yielded a negative result.'[3]

I argue that when we actually look at the examples which Lamerton gives of 'good medicine', we will see that the judgements and decisions they involve do not, after all, differ *in kind* from the judgements and decisions which would be involved in the practice of euthanasia. It is not the case, in other words, that different *types* of judgement are involved; it is not the case that we can make this particular contrast between judgements which are medical and judgements which are moral. There is a distinction between purely clinical judgements and moral judgements, but the judgements contained in Dr Lamerton's examples are none of them purely clinical judgements. It does not follow that he is not entitled to call them medical judgements; the point is, rather, that their being medical judgements is not incompatible with their also being moral judgements. This is not merely an academic point; as we shall see, it has implications for the question of *whose* judgements they should be.

THE RIGHT TIME TO DIE

Before I look at the examples Lamerton gives, I want to say something very briefly about this idea of 'the right time to die', as we might find it in a non-medical context.

Suppose I say of someone 'He died at the right time'; what do I mean? I might mean one of a number of things. What I actually mean can only be determined if the context in which the remark is made is supplied, and in some detail. I might mean, for example, that he died before what truly mattered to him disappeared from his life – for example, his capacity for listening to music, for intellectual inquiry, or for hang-gliding. Or I might mean that he has escaped knowledge which would have devastated his life; the knowledge perhaps that his life's work had been in vain or that his children had died or brought dishonour and shame to his family. One can escape all sorts of disasters by being fortunate enough to die before they occur. Thus death is not always a disaster.

When the murder of King Duncan is discovered, Macbeth, his murderer, says in feigned grief: 'Had I but died an hour before this chance, I had lived a blessed time.'[4] Macbeth is actually right in what he says; this shows that among the disasters we can escape by dying at the right time are moral disasters. Had Macbeth died before he killed Duncan, he would have escaped the moral disaster of becoming a murderer.

Of course, dying at the right time is not always a matter of escaping disasters, moral or otherwise. I might say of someone, 'She died at the right time', meaning that she had accomplished her purposes in life and was content to leave it. The words of Simeon in the Temple are a good illustration of this: 'Now lettest thou thy servant depart in peace according to Thy word, for mine eyes have seen Thy salvation. . . .' There is now no reason to stay.

I will resist the temptation to pile up examples of this kind; those I have given are important, however, because they display two things: first, the need for a context if we are to speak meaningfully of the right time to die, and second, the essential role within any context we may mention of values in a broad sense. It is these values that give a claim, that someone has died at the right time, the precise meaning or the precise significance that it has. To put the point in general terms, something good has been accomplished and/or something bad escaped or averted; in the examples I gave, for the dead person himself or herself. It could, of course, be for others or also for others.

What has all this got to do with medicine, with the medical judgement that, for a particular patient, the right time to die has come? Simply this: that here too we have of necessity the idea of some good achieved or some evil escaped or averted. Here too, then, we have values; we cannot get away from them.

THE MEDICAL CONTEXT

Let us look at three of the examples Dr Lamerton gives. I remind the reader that I am not medically trained and I know nothing more about these cases than I have read in Dr Lamerton's book.

1 If a man has lost a large slice of brain in a road accident but still goes on breathing he should not be given antibiotics to prevent infection of the wound. It is a legitimate medical judgement to decide that it is not in the interest of the patient to resuscitate him.[5]

2 When a total bowel obstruction develops in a patient with widespread abdominal cancer and the surgeon cannot operate

further, this should be seen as a terminal event. Antispasmodics combined with sedation are much kinder at this stage than drip and suck treatment which merely ensures that the patient takes three weeks to die instead of three days.[6]

3 Having come slowly to terms with her family, her disease and finally with God, [Mrs P.] died at the right time of pneumonia, which we did not try to treat.[7]

I suggest that with respect to all three of these examples the role of values within them is both crucial and obvious, if we think about it.

In the first example what determines the decision not to use antibiotics is *the interests of the patient*. Any judgement about where a patient's interests lie is a value judgement; here, one based on the assessment of the kind or quality of life this patient would have were he to go on living. Quality of life judgements are value judgements. Furthermore, the giving of priority to the interests of the patient over any other factors involved is itself a matter of value.

In the second example, as in the third, what is at stake is a particular conception of what it is to die well. The emphasis in the second example is possibly on physical factors, for example the presence or absence of pain; the emphasis in the third is on psychological and spiritual factors. All these factors are involved in the conception which Lamerton has, and which I believe many others share, of *the good death*, of what it is to die well.

I do not wish to criticise any of those decisions; I want to point out that they all involve moral judgements. There is nothing wrong with this – the fact is that without moral values there could be no practice of medicine at all. The practice of medicine must involve more than medical science.

It is this point which the above examples illustrate. I shall now enlarge upon it in response to certain objections which might be levelled against what I have said so far.

One objection may turn on the alleged significance of the distinction between 'killing' and 'letting die'. It might be said that when doctors 'let die', as in the above examples, they are merely *acknowledging certain facts*; compare what Lamerton himself says in the passage noted above about a 'test' or 'trial of therapy'. The judgements involved are therefore not moral in character as I have said, but scientific or clinical. There is here no decision which goes beyond the facts, in the way in which a decision to kill would go beyond the facts.

What are the facts which, on this view, a doctor merely acknowledges when he withdraws or withholds treatment? An obvious answer would seem to be: the fact that the patient cannot be cured, and that therefore treatment would be pointless or futile: that is to say, *it would do no good*. We need to look more closely, however, at this way of speaking; for it is *ambiguous*. The ambiguity is a crucial one in the context of the present discussion.

It might be said in certain circumstances that giving a particular drug (for example) to a patient *would do no good*, meaning that it would *have no effect at all upon the patient's condition*. In these circumstances, it seems to me, 'it would do no good' *is* a scientific or clinical judgement, and we could speak of the doctor as 'merely acknowledging the facts'. There is simply nothing to be done, either through this method of treatment or – let us suppose – any other.

In other circumstances, however, 'it would do no good' might mean not 'it would have no effect' but 'the effect it would have *is best avoided*'. That is, the treatment under discussion would do something, but not something good, not something that morally ought to be done.

This is precisely what is being said in the first and second of the examples quoted from Lamerton's book. On the first, administering antibiotics *would* prevent infection of the wound in the patient's brain, and would therefore (I take it) assist in resuscitation. What Lamerton is saying is that it would be better in these circumstances if a resuscitation were not brought about, better from the standpoint of the patient's *interests*. This, as I have said above, is not a clinical or scientific judgement, but a moral judgement. Facts are, of course, relevant to this judgement, but it cannot be reduced to a statement of the facts. It is made in response to the facts, certainly, and one might therefore call it an acknowledgement of them. It is not 'merely' an acknowledgement of them, however, because it is the values which Lamerton brings to this situation which determine for him the form which a *proper* acknowledgement must take.

The same sort of point must be made about the second example, that of the patient with terminal cancer who develops a total bowel obstruction. This patient's life cannot be saved, but it is clear from what Lamerton himself says that it can be prolonged for some weeks by the drip and suck method of treatment. It is not the case, in other words, that this treatment would be futile or pointless, in the sense of having no effect. What is the case, Lamerton is saying, is that the effect it would have is a *morally* undesirable one. His view is that it would not be *kind* to prolong the patient's life in this way. This is quite plainly a moral judgement, and not a clinical or scientific one; it cannot be reduced to a value-free description of what the consequences of the drip and suck method here would be. Once again, it is the values which Lamerton brings to the situation which determine for him what is to count as a proper response to or acknowledgement of the facts contained in such a description.

It is easier to see this point if we consider the way in which someone with quite different values might respond to the situation Lamerton describes. Lamerton says that it is not the duty of a physician to prolong life for as long as he can, irrespective of the condition the patient is in, and most of us, I am sure, would agree with him. Suppose, however, that we were Parsees, who believe (I am told) that death is a victory of evil over good. If we did hold this belief, and were to take it seriously, we might well insist that it is the duty of a doctor to prolong life at any cost; in which case the drip and suck method of treatment is the one we would advocate in the situation under discussion.

It is not the case, then, that when doctors 'let die', as opposed to kill, they are merely acknowledging certain facts; indeed, one would surely not speak of 'letting die' at all if there were really *nothing* that could be done to prolong at least the life in question. When one 'lets die' one *chooses* to do so, and this choice is a *moral* one. In that respect it is in the same category as a choice to kill; it is not the case that the former is 'medical' and only the latter 'moral'.

It may be said in response to this point that if it is correct then the judgements of which Lamerton, for example, approves are no more within the remit of medical practice than those of which he disapproves. In other words, doctors as doctors should *neither* kill *nor* let die until they are told to do so; since these are both *moral* choices they should be made by people whose business it is to make them, whoever they are – the patient's relatives and friends, perhaps.

The trouble with this response, I would argue, is that it is destructive of the whole practice of medicine itself, which necessarily involves more than medical science. Medical science must be applied in a human context, and values in a broad sense – aims, goals, purposes, priorities, conceptions of the good – are necessary to its application. The *practice* of medicine must be imbued with certain values, it cannot be value-free; and one of the values central to it is the one to which Lamerton is appealing in all of the examples he gives – that of the well-being or interests of the patient. Thus, in saying that a decision to let die is a moral decision, one that refers to certain values, I am not denying that it can be called a medical decision. It could be a medical decision; so could a decision to kill. If we have regard to the values which enter into medical practice, we can see that a judgement can be *both* moral and medical. It is not the case that if it is one it cannot also be the other.

This point, that the practice of medicine cannot be value-free, might be easier to grasp if we think not in terms of medicine but in terms of health care. The concept of health care is overtly value-laden; there could be no credible supposition that the judgements and decisions involved in caring for health might be all value-free. In caring for people's health we are caring for people, and this implies the centrality of their interests in the choices and decisions that we make.

WHOSE DECISIONS?

There is, however, this much truth in the second objection referred to above: decisions to kill, or to let die, are not ones which only doctors have the competence to make. Lamerton seems to imply otherwise; his failure to see that certain medical judgements are also moral judgements brings him dangerously close to presenting them not as matters for experienced doctors *among others*, but as matters for experienced doctors *alone*. He speaks as if decisions to withdraw or withhold treatment involve the exercise of special expertise, the sort of special expertise which doctors and no one else possess. It is for them, he implies, to make decisions of this sort and other people must simply accept the decisions that they make.

It is true, of course, that doctors – or at least persons with medical training – are the experts as far as the relevant clinical facts are concerned. In the case of the cancer patient referred to above, for example, only a medically trained person would know what exactly had happened to the patient's bowel, and how this might be dealt with. As far as *moral* judgements are concerned, however, there are no *experts* at all; and this applies to the medico-moral judgements with which this chapter is concerned.

Consider the cancer patient again. If there is a choice to be made here, as there would seem to be, it is not one which only his doctor, or other medically trained person, is competent to make. Given the facts, the question is: should this person be allowed to die in three days, or should his life be prolonged for three weeks? This, as we have seen, is a moral question, and it follows that the patient himself, his relatives, his friends, his nurses are as competent as his doctor to answer it. (Indeed, it is clear that some of these people may have a greater right to answer it than the doctor does.)

This point, at last, brings us back to the central concern of this paper; for it applies equally to another question: should this person have to take three days to die, let alone three weeks? Lamerton himself regards hastening a patient's death – that is to say, killing a patient – as morally out of the question. I have not considered the arguments he gives in support of this position (in chapter 9 of *Care of the Dying*), nor have I argued myself either for or against euthanasia. I have been concerned only with his attempt, as I construe it, to place euthanasia outside the remit of medical practice. I have argued that this attempt does not succeed. Whatever answer is given to the question posed above, and whoever should take the ultimate responsibility for giving this answer, Lamerton has failed to show that doctors and other health carers exceed their brief by raising it.[8]

NOTES

1 Lamerton, R., *Care of the Dying*, London: Priory Press, 1973.
2 ibid., p. 75.
3 ibid., p. 89.
4 William Shakespeare, *Macbeth*, Act II, Scene 3.
5 Lamerton, op. cit., pp. 90–1.
6 ibid., p. 39.
7 ibid., p. 77.
8 An earlier version of this paper was presented at two conferences on terminal care organised in London and Wrexham by the Marie Curie Foundation. I am grateful to all those who contributed to its discussion, especially Revd Rod Cosh. I am also grateful to Dr Geoffrey Hunt for his written comments.

Chapter 12

Nurse time as a scarce health care resource

Donna Dickenson

For a very long time discussion about scarce health care resource allocation was limited to allocation of *medical* resources, and the paradigmatic case was kidney transplants. Two sorts of criteria emerged from this debate: clinical – who is the most 'savable'? – and social – who is the most 'worth saving'? Although writers on the subject pointed out that medical criteria were often thinly veiled social ones, by and large they opted for one or the other.

In this chapter I shall suggest that their narrow focus on medical resources prevented these authors from seeing that there are many cases – perhaps even the majority – in which neither clinical nor social criteria work. The allocation of nursing time as a scarce health care resource may have to be made on quite different grounds, and everyday decisions about that dilemma far outnumber the more attention-getting cases about organ transplants. In discussing nurse time as a scarce resource, I shall go on to argue that the two principles to be respected are nurse autonomy and randomisation.

MEDICAL AND SOCIAL

In the case of organ transplants and dialysis allocation, there have been many vociferous claims that clinical criteria are to be preferred because they are objective. For example, the United States National Organ Transplant Task Force recommended medical standards as the fairest and most rational in its 1986 report. The aim is to 'maximize graft and patient survival and quality of life'.[1] But what constitutes the most medically 'correct' choice is ambivalent. The most 'savable' in terms of prognosis is unlikely to be either the neediest or 'illest' in terms of diagnosis – a point to which I shall return later in discussing a fictional case study about the allocation of nurse time.

Nor are medical criteria as objective as is sometimes claimed. A purely medical set of standards for organ allocation turns out to benefit whites disproportionately, for example.[2] Because histo-compatibility makes a successful graft more likely, the Task Force suggested the medical benefit rule of a six-HLA antigen match and no mismatches. But it turns out to be harder to obtain six antigen matches in Afro-Caribbeans because their donor pool is smaller in the USA (or in Britain) than the white one. As Robert Veatch puts it, 'This means that a policy that gives priority to the best tissue matches will be a policy that gives priority to whites.'[3]

No one is claiming that a medical standard for allocation of scarce resources deliberately tries to penalise already disadvantaged groups. But that is frequently its effect. In the same year in which the US Task Force brought out its recommendations, an infant heart transplant candidate, 'Baby Jesse', was refused the procedure on 'medical' grounds.[4] Although he met the preliminary clinical criteria, his parents were unmarried teenagers with a criminal history and drug abuse problems. They were judged incapable of providing the necessary follow-up procedures, such as punctual administration of immuno-suppressive medications.

About the same time, in a case at the Churchill Hospital in Oxford, a vagrant patient's dialysis was terminated because he was judged unable to follow the diet and other requirements for success-ful treatment. Although these were presented as purely medical criteria, the case caused an outcry, particularly among the hospital's nursing staff. Well-educated and affluent patients or parents have the best chances of looking after themselves or their children properly, of course. To maximise the chances of a successful graft, and avoid 'wasting' a heart or kidney, the medical model would suggest concentrating the resource among the well educated and affluent.

Medical criteria shade over into social ones, and social criteria have had a very bad press since the Seattle 'God' committee closed down operations. This body was set up in the early 1960s with apparently laudable aims: to reassure the community that doctors were not playing God, ironically enough. It, too, claimed to be able to make choices objectively: its director, Dr Belding Scribner, hoped 'to represent the community and assure that choices are made objectively and without outside pressure'.[5] Although the committee did set some medical guidelines, it was primarily concerned with social variables in drawing up its recommendations for allocation of kidney transplants: net worth, marital status, church membership, Scout leadership, psychological stability and present or potential future income. Decisions were made in secret, and no criteria for individual decisions were published. Most criticism at the time – attacks which, combined with members' feelings of guilt, were virulent enough to close the committee down – focused on the class bias of these criteria: 'the bourgeoisie saving the bourgeoisie'.[6]

Rules favouring high earners will also discriminate against women, however. The committee was willing to give preference to a non-earning housewife with small children, but once these hostages to fortune were grown, older women would have had to take their chances – rigged chances.

THE CASE OF MRS ROBERTSON

In contrast to the thirty-year-old debate about medical versus social criteria in the allocation of organ transplants, discussion of nurse time as a scarce health care resource is still relatively new. I want to show that looking at the allocation of scarce resources from the particular viewpoint of nursing time makes both the usual sorts of criteria look strangely irrelevant.

Robert Veatch and Sara Fry have developed a fictional example of a nurse who is confronted with the entirely typical case in which her duty is not to the patient, but to patients in the plural.[7] On a medical-surgical nursing care unit, night nurse Clora Bingham has four needy patients. Mrs Robertson is an 83-year-old woman who is dying and semi-comatose, in need of a suctioning procedure every fifteen to twenty minutes to prevent a mucous plug from blocking her bronchi and causing respiratory failure. Mr Jablowski, 47, was admitted for observation and has had several bloody bowel movements. Mr Hanson, 52, is a newly diagnosed diabetic with unstable blood sugar levels who needs frequent vital sign checks and is getting intravenous insulin. The fourth patient, 35-year-old Mr Manfra, has no immediate medical needs but has been suicidal in the past. Fears that he might now repeat his suicidal behaviour have been heightened: he learned today that he has inoperable cancer of the spine.

It seems unlikely that Clora Bingham can actually give all four patients equal amounts of her time, or that, if she could, this would be the right thing to do. If she has to suction Mrs Robertson every fifteen to twenty minutes, she will be unable to give Mr Manfra the length of time for a talk which he might need. She will effectively do him no good at all if she rushes off in the middle of one of his sentences, and perhaps even some harm: he may become all the more depressed and angry. It looks very much as if her time is effectively indivisible, just like a kidney – although a first reaction to the issue of nurse time as a scarce resource is to say that it is divisible, unlike the kidney.

On either clinical or social utility criteria, Mrs Robertson seems the least 'important', although her condition is the most critical. She cannot be saved, and she has less 'useful' potential life span to contribute to society than any of the three younger patients. Assuming for the moment that no negligence suit or disciplinary action would result, should Clora Bingham forget about Mrs Robertson?

That this appears quite unacceptable says something uncomplimentary about clinical and social utility criteria. It shows the extent to which discussion of scarce resources has been too strictly medical, in terms of organ transplants and dialysis. Thinking in terms of the nurse's decision is a useful counterweight. How could she continue to view herself as a responsible person if she left Mrs Robertson to die unattended?

Nurses have been found to be able to cope with a patient's death most easily when they can tell themselves, with justice, that nothing more could have been done. Their peace of mind seems to depend on it. In interviewing nurses on a coronary care unit, David Field found that there was surprisingly little sense of 'failure' when a patient died, so long as the nurses were sure that they had done everything possible to stave off the death. Although the purpose of the unit was to prevent death, and nurses might have been expected to feel remorse when they failed to save a patient, good staffing, ward organisation and technology did indeed give backing to the nurses' view that those who could be saved were being saved. The nurses, all qualified, were legally covered to give drugs and instigate life-saving treatment even if no doctor was present. Deaths were infrequent (about 7.5 per cent of admissions), and nurses better able to cope with them than junior doctors, interestingly. One nurse's comments are indicative:

> We're dealing with people on a fairly narrow range of medical problems, and usually we know whether we can do anything constructive in a situation or whether it's hopeless, and so we're

not left with that guilt feeling that I experienced sometimes as a student of not knowing whether there might have been anything more that I could have done, because usually you say, 'Well, we did everything that could possible have been done in the situation and there was nothing I could have done to avert what happened.'[8]

It would be wrong, and probably psychologically intolerable, for the nurse to omit a procedure which she knows to be necessary for keeping a patient alive, even if by some miraculous chance Mrs Robertson survived despite Clora Bingham missing one or more of her suctioning times. (This assumes that Mrs Robertson has not signed a living will or given some other indication before entering the semi-comatose state that she wanted nothing further done for her; and that she is not suffering so greatly that moral questions about prolonging her agony would arise even in the absence of a living will.)

How will Clora Bingham feel if she devotes the maximum time to Mrs Robertson and Mr Manfra manages to commit suicide? In a sense suicide is Mr Manfra's own project, not hers, and an extreme view of patients' rights might stress that it was his free choice. But an initial suicidal reaction to diagnosis of inoperable cancer is sometimes followed by determination to live the remaining life to the full. Could Clora Bingham be sure that Mr Manfra might not have changed his mind, given a bit of her time? Clearly not, but she can be much more sure about what will happen to Mrs Robertson if she misses her suctioning procedure. Mrs Robertson is almost certain to die without the treatment, and to die during Clora Bingham's shift. There is no equivalent level of certainty with Mr Manfra.

Whatever the odds, if Mr Manfra commits suicide Clora Bingham will doubtless feel deep regret. But there is no reason for her to experience remorse and guilt, which would have to do with some moral failure of hers. Mr Manfra's suicide is nothing to do with such a failure: it is ultimately his decision. And she is much more likely to feel guilty about Mrs Robertson's death if she knows there was something she could have done about it. I would argue that Mrs Robertson has the first claim on Clora Bingham's time, not as a result of qualities inherent in the patient – either the possibility of clinical benefit or greater 'social utility' – but because of the nurse's own moral sensibilities, which are infringed by letting Mrs Robertson die just to follow medical utility criteria.

RANDOMISATION

Assuming that any time remains after Mrs Robertson's suctioning procedures have been carried out, how should Clora Bingham divide it? I want to suggest that she should give serious thought to a third principle which has sometimes been suggested to decide who gets the kidney or the expensive operation, but which has generally had less influence than medical or social criteria: randomisation.[9] Again, using the example of nurse time as the scarce resource gives a different result.

In relation to allocation of kidneys, a minority of writers have argued for randomisation, or equalisation of chances. No patient is to get the kidney on grounds of better clinical prognosis or greater 'social utility'; everyone is given equal chances through the device of a 'lottery', or, in practice, through a first-come-first-served system. This model sounds impractical, but it is described as being the basis of the Italian system of kidney allocation.[10] Italian doctors refuse to use lack of clinical merit as a criterion, because patients do not choose to suffer from serious conditions: 'Why, after all, should their shorter lives be measured against lives that would have been longer from no merit of their own?'[11]

In contexts other than kidney allocation, lotteries have sometimes been held to be the only fair and 'objective' way of deciding between claims to scarce resources. Freund has said,

> The more nearly total is the estimate to be made of an individual, and the more nearly the consequence determines life and death, the more unfit the judgement becomes for human reckoning. . . . Randomness as a moral principle deserves serious study.[12]

The most gripping example of this policy is the case of *U.S.* v. *Holmes* (1841), in which the presiding judge ruled that a surviving crew member, Holmes, should not have collaborated with his mates in devising and implementing social criteria for deciding who among a shipwreck's survivors must be thrown off a lifeboat in order to lighten its load. Despite his counsel's contention that the crew's method of selection – 'not to part man and wife, and not to throw over any woman' – was more humane than drawing straws, Holmes was convicted of unlawful homicide. (In fact the crew members failed to prevent female deaths: two sisters jumped overboard to drown with their brother, who was among the fourteen men jettisoned.) In the judge's opinion, only casting lots would have been a remedy which the law could sanction: 'In no other way than this or some like way are those having equal rights put on an equal footing, and in no other way is it possible to guard against partiality and oppression, violence and conflict.'[13] In the Clora Bingham example, we are also concerned with 'those having equal rights' being 'put on an equal footing'. But we can modify the general principle of randomisation to this case, which is really more about equalisation of chances for those having equal rights. In the Holmes case, there was no way to divide up the precious good, the place in the lifeboat: it was all or nothing. I argued earlier that the nurse's time was actually more indivisible than it looked at first. But now that we have taken care of the prime constraint on her time, Mrs Robertson, Clora's remaining time could be divided up equally, to give 'those having equal rights' – the remaining three patients – equal chances. The principle behind this is egalitarianism, the same principle that lies behind randomisation, but the application of the principle in this case calls for equalisation.

For Clora Bingham to divide her time equally among the remaining three patients, in accordance with the principle of egalitarianism, should be feasible, I think, though there are still more problems in giving Mr Manfra what he needs than there are for the other two men. Let us assume that Mr Hanson's vital sign checks need to be carried out less frequently than the suctioning procedure did for Mrs Robertson. Say that as an adult-onset diabetic, he is perhaps less likely to lapse into coma than a young patient might be.[14] If the checks and observations for Mr Jablowski and Mr Hanson allow substantial intervals, Clora Bingham may well be able to give Mr Manfra some uninterrupted time for a talk. There is no reason why she has to equalise her time mechanically: the principle does not require precisely five minutes for each of the three patients every fifteen minutes.

Clearly if any of the three men die, Clora Bingham will feel grief and regret, but she would not necessarily feel remorse or decide that her action in apportioning her residual time equally among them was wrong. Dividing her remaining time equally overall will be Clora Bingham's way of 'getting it right' whatever the outcome for the three remaining patients, I think. It will also spare her a lengthy weighing-up of the three individual patients' precise claims to portions of her time – making the scarce resource of her time still scarcer.

Equalising the nurse's time, once the urgent claims of the dying patient are met, corresponds to the principle of casting lots among the remaining patients.

AGE AND AGEISM

Robert Veatch proposes a modified form of randomised allocation for organ transplants: 'People in equal need of an organ ought to have an equal shot at it even if one potential recipient would be more likely to make a socially worthwhile contribution.'[15] But Veatch also wants to weight in age, the obvious objection to randomising nursing time. A 90-year-old might be seen to 'deserve' less of the nurse's precious time than a younger person, if benefit is measured in terms of years of life which the nurse can add.

But we have already seen that ignoring the urgent claims of the oldest person in the fictionalised example, Mrs Robertson, was deeply counter-intuitive. Clora Bingham's moral autonomy and peace of mind depended on her doing all she could for the dying Mrs Robertson. For less acute cases, however, should a nurse divide her time according to the age of patients? After all, if there is only one dialysis machine or kidney available, and a choice must be made between giving it to an 80-year-old and a 20-year-old, most people find the answer obvious enough.

However, the nurse owes a duty of care to both the 80-year-old and the 20-year-old, if both are patients on her ward. Does she somehow owe a little more duty to the 20-year-old? The criterion of age is a very slippery slope. John Harris is suspicious of automatic preference for younger patients, which he calls a form of ageism; but even he sets a 'fair innings' standard of 70 years, the statistically average life-span.[16] No one over that age is to be allowed the scarce medical resource in preference to someone younger. (Harris, in common with most authors until recently, does not discuss nurse time.)

As with all criteria open to the 'slippery slope' objection, the age limit of 70 raises some obvious absurdities. A patient who presents herself for treatment at a dialysis centre on her seventy-first birthday would be turned away, whereas she would have been treated if she had arrived a day earlier. It is not at all clear what is so magical about 70. If years of life which the health care professional could add are the criterion, any arbitrary age limit will be less effective than a complete analysis of the patient's life-style and clinical prognosis.

But that will shade into social criteria again: a 71-year-old who can afford the proper diet and is well educated about healthy living will be a better bet than a 70-year-old with none of these advantages. And the first patient is more likely to be middle class.

Is 70 the magic age because it is somehow the 'norm'? But women live on average six or seven years longer than men: a cut-off point of 70 will disadvantage women and advantage men. In both cases, the supposedly impartial age limit turns out to reinforce existing social inequality. And because people in modern Western societies do normally live to a statistical average of 70 says nothing at all about whether they should live till 70. To argue otherwise is a form of the naturalistic fallacy, the common assumption being that a form of behaviour which is natural is also morally right.

It might be argued that the 71-year-old has already enjoyed 'a good life'. In Veatch's view, justice as fairness demands that,

> persons be given an opportunity to have well-being over a lifetime equal to that of others. This means that infants, who have had no opportunity for well-being, would get a higher priority than older persons who have had many good years of life.[17]

But what if the years have not been good, or are just becoming so? If life is good, it does not necessarily become any less sweet with age, assuming that the patient is not in pain or distress which cannot be palliated. If it has not been good – and Veatch tends to assume that it has – a last chance at happiness is being denied. On this argument, we would always give preference to the youngest person, and Mr Manfra would get the bulk of Clora Bingham's time, leaving Mrs Robertson to die unattended. That this goes against the grain shows how little nurse time – and nurse autonomy – have counted until recently in discussion about allocation of scarce resources.

CONCLUSION

The ethical dilemmas faced by nurses in dividing the valuable resource of their available time have been largely invisible in the literature on scarce resources, which has been medically orientated. I hope that this chapter will have gone a little way towards rectifying that omission, even for those who disagree with its conclusions. These are that the guiding principle should be randomisation (equalisation) – which respects patients as persons by putting them all on an equal level – and nurse autonomy to decide otherwise in difficult cases such as dying patients – which respects nurses as moral agents.

NOTES

1 United States Department of Health and Human Services, Task Force on Organ Transplantation, *Organ Transplantation: Issues and Recommendations*, Washington, D.C.: Department of Health and Human Services, 1986, p. 87.

2 Veatch, R. M., *Death, Dying and the Biological Revolution: Our Last Quest for Responsibility*, New Haven: Yale University Press, 1989, revised edn, p. 207.

3 ibid.

4 The US Task Force did not want to exclude medically suitable applicants because they lacked social support. It therefore suggested that social service agencies should make up any deficiencies. How realistic this recommendation is must be open to doubt.

5 Calabresi, G. and Bobbitt, P., *Tragic Choices*, New York: W. W. Norton & Company, 1978, footnote 110, p. 232.

6 Sanders, D. and Dukeminier, J., 'Medical Advance and Legal Lag', *U.C.L.A. Law Review*, 1968, vol. 15, pp. 377–8. For further critical discussion of the Seattle 'God' Committee, see Calabresi and Bobbitt, op. cit., pp. 187–8, and footnotes 111–12, p. 233.

7 Veatch, R. M. and Fry, S. T., *Case Studies in Nursing Ethics*, Philadelphia: J.B. Lippincott Co., 1987, case 23, 'Allocating Nursing Time According to Benefit', pp. 84 ff.

8 Field, D., *Nursing the Dying*, London: Tavistock/Routledge, 1989, p. 78. That nurses were best able to cope with a patient's death when they could justifiably feel that they had done everything possible was also reported in Glaser, B. G. and Strauss, A. L., *Awareness of Dying*, Chicago: Aldine, 1965.

9 Randomisation is widely used as a principle for dividing up groups of subjects in clinical trials, of course, but very rarely in allocating scarce health care resources.

10 In Calabresi and Bobbitt, op. cit., pp. 182 ff.

11 ibid, p. 182.

12 Freund, P. A., 'Introduction: Ethical Aspects of Experimentation with Human Subjects', *Daedalus*, Spring 1969, p. xiii. A similar argument is made in Katz, A., 'Process Design for Selection of Haemodialysis and Organ Transplant Recipients', *Buffalo Law Review*, 1973, vol. 22, and in Ramsey, P., *The Patient as Person: Explorations in Medical Ethics*, New Haven, Conn. Yale University Press, 1970, pp. 259–66. However, Katz ultimately proposes that the lottery be limited to a pool of clinically suitable applicants, tempering randomisation with medical criteria. This approach is also taken by Childress, J. F., 'Who Shall Live When Not All Can Live?', in S. Gorovitz *et al.*, *Moral Problems in Medicine*, Englewood Cliffs, N. J. Prentice-Hall, 1983, 2nd edition; Outka, G., 'Social Justice and Equal Access to Health Care,' *Journal of Religious Ethics*, 1974, vol. 2, pp. 11–32; and Green, R. M., 'Health Care and

Justice in Contract Theory Perspective,' in Veatch, R. M. and Branson, R. (eds), *Ethics and Health Policy*, Cambridge, Mass.: Ballinger Publishing, 1976, pp. 111–26.

13 *U.S.* v. *Holmes*, 26 Fed. Case 360.

14 Armstrong, M. E., *et al.* (eds), *McGraw-Hill Handbook of Clinical Nursing*, Tokyo: McGraw-Hill Kogashuka, 1979, pp. 684–5.

15 Veatch, op. cit., 1989, p. 206.

16 Harris, J., *The Value of Life: An Introduction to Medical Ethics*, London: Routledge & Kegan Paul, 1985, pp. 88 ff.

17 Veatch, op. cit., 1989, pp. 204–5.

Bibliography

Alderson, P., 'Trust in Informed Consent', *IME Bulletin* (Institute of Medical Ethics), 1988, no. 40, pp. 17–19.
—— *Children's Consent to Surgery*, Milton Keynes: Open University Press, 1993.
Altschul, A., *Patient–Nurse Interaction: A Study of Interaction Patterns in Acute Psychiatric Wards*, Edinburgh: Churchill Livingstone, 1972.
Armstrong, M. E., Dickason, E. J., Howe, J. *et al.* (eds), *McGraw-Hill Handbook of Clinical Nursing*, New York: McGraw-Hill, 1979.
Askham, J., *A Review of Research on Falls Among Elderly People*, London: Age Concern Institute of Gerontology, King's College, London, 1990.
Athlin, E. and Norberg, A., 'Care-givers' Attitudes to and Interpretations of the Behaviour of Severely Demented Patients during Feeding in a Patient Assignment Care System', *International Journal of Nursing Studies*, 1987, vol. 24 (2), pp. 145–53.
Bancroft, J., *Human Sexuality and its Problems*, London: Churchill Livingstone, 1989.
Beauchamp, T. L. and Childress, J. F., *Principles of Biomedical Ethics*, 3rd edn, New York: Oxford University Press, 1989.
Bebeau, M. J. and Brabeck, M. M., 'Integrating Care and Justice Issues in Professional Moral Education: A Gender Perspective', *Journal of Moral Education*, 1987, vol. 16 (3), pp. 189–203.
Bercusson, B., *The Employment Protection (Consolidation) Act 1978*, London: Sweet & Maxwell, 1979.
Bergman, R., 'Accountability: Definitions and Dimensions', *International Nursing Review*, 1981, vol. 28 (2), pp. 53–9.
Blackburn, M. C., Bax, M. C. O., Strehlow, C. and Hunt, Y., 'Sexual Knowledge and Experiences of Young Adults with Spina Bifida and Hydrocephalus', *Research Report for the Association of Spina Bifida and Hydrocephalus*, 1994 (in press).
Blackburn, M. C. and Bax, M. C. O., 'Sex Education Provision for Young Adults with Spina Bifida and/or Hydrocephalus: An Evaluation of a Pilot Training Video', *European Journal of Paediatric Surgery*, 1992, vol. 2 (Supp. 1), pp. 39–40.

Bond, S., 'Nurses' Communications with Cancer Patients', in J. Wilson-Barnett (ed.), *Nursing Research : Ten Studies in Patient Care*, Chichester: John Wiley & Sons, 1983, pp. 57–79.

Booth, W., 'A Cry for Help in the Wilderness', *The Health Service Journal*, 14 February 1991, vol. 101, pp. 26–7.

Brazier, M., *Medicine, Patients and the Law*, Harmondsworth: Penguin Books, 1987.

Byrne, D. J., Napier, A. and Cuschieri, A., 'How Informed is Signed Consent?' *British Medical Journal*, 1988, vol. 296, pp. 839–40.

Byrne, P. (ed.), *Health, Rights and Resources: King's College Studies 1987–88*, London: King Edward's Hospital Fund for London, 1988.

Calabresi, G. and Bobbitt, P., *Tragic Choices*, New York: W. W. Norton & Company, 1978.

Callahan, J. C. (ed.), *Ethical Issues in Professional Life*, New York and Oxford: Oxford University Press, 1988.

Card, C., 'Women's Voices and Ethical Ideals: Must we Mean What we Say?', *Ethics*, 1988, vol. 98, pp. 125–35.

Carson, D. and Montgomery, J., *Nursing and the Law*, London: Macmillan, 1989.

Centres for Disease Control, 'Revision of the CDC Surveillance Case Definition of Acquired Immuno-deficiency Syndrome', *Morbidity and Mortality Weekly Report*, 1987, vol. 36, Supplement No. 1S.

Childress, J. F., 'Who Shall Live When Not All Can Live?', in Gorovitz, S. *et al.*, *Moral Problems in Medicine*, Englewood Cliffs : Prentice-Hall, 2nd edn, 1983.

Chrystie, I. L., Palmer, S. J., Kenney, A., Banatvala, J. E., 'HIV Seroprevalence among Women Attending Antenatal Clinics in London', *The Lancet*, vol. 33 (8 February 1992) p. 364.

Cox, C., *Sociology, An Introduction for Nurses, Midwives and Health Visitors*, London: Butterworth, 1983.

Creighton, H., 'Decisions on Food and Fluid in Life Sustaining Measures', *Nursing Management*, 1984, vol. 15 (6), pp. 47–9 and vol. 15 (7), pp. 54–6.

Croft, S. and Beresford, P., 'User Involvement, Citizenship and Social Policy', *Critical Social Policy*, 1989, vol. 26, pp. 5–18.

Culver, C. M. and Gert, B., *Philosophy in Medicine*, Oxford: Oxford University Press, 1982.

Curtin, L. and Flaherty, M. J. (eds), *Nursing Ethics: Theories and Pragmatics*, Englewood Cliffs, USA: Prentice-Hall, 1982.

Davidson, B., Vander Laan, R., Hirschfeld, M., Norberg, A., Pitman, E. and Ju Ying, L., 'Ethical Reasoning Associated with the Feeding of Terminally Ill Cancer Patients. An International Perspective', *Cancer Nursing*, 1990, vol. 13 (5), pp. 286–92.

De Selincourt K., 'A Breach of Trust?' *Nursing Times*, 1992, vol. 88 (11), p. 19.

Dean, D. J., *Manpower Solutions*, London: Royal College of Nursing, 1987.

Department of Health and Human Services (USA), Task Force on Organ Transplantation, *Organ Transplantation: Issues and Recommendations*, Washington, DC: Department of Health and Human Services, 1986.

Department of Health, *Working for Patients* (CM555), London: Department of Health 1989 (and eight Working Papers).

—— *A Guide to Consent for Examination and Treatment*, Heywood, Lancs.: Department of Health, 1990.

—— *Local Research Ethics Committees*, Heywood, Lancs.: Department of Health 1991 (HSG(91)5).

Department of Health and Social Security (DHSS), *Report of the Committee on Nursing*, London: DHSS, 1972.

—— *Code of Practice, Mental Health Act 1983*, London: DHSS, 1990.

Dimond, B., *Legal Aspects of Nursing*, London: Prentice Hall, 1990.

Dixon, E., *The Theatre Nurse and the Law*, London: Croom Helm, 1984.

Dock, S., 'The Relation of the Nurse to the Doctor and the Doctor to the Nurse', *American Journal of Nursing*, 1917, vol. 17, p. 394.

Dorner, S., 'Sexual Interest and Activities in Adolescents with Spina Bifida', *Journal of Child Psychology and Psychiatry*, 1977, vol. 18, pp. 229–37.

Downie, R. S. and Calman, K. C., *Healthy Respect: Ethics in Health Care*, London: Faber & Faber, 1987.

Dresser, R., 'When Patients Resist Feeding: Medical, Ethical and Legal Considerations', *Journal of the American Geriatrics Society*, 1985, vol. 33 (11), pp. 790–4.

Dunne, L. M., 'Quality Assurance: Methods of Measurement', *The Professional Nurse*, March 1987, p. 188.

Edser, P. and Ward, G., 'Sexuality, Sex and Spina Bifida', in Bannister, C. M. and Tew, B., *Current Concepts in Spina Bifida and Hydrocephalus*, London: McKeith Press and Blackwell Scientific, 1991.

Faulder, C., *Whose Body is it? The Troubling Issue of Informed Consent*, London: Virago Press, 1985.

Faulkner, A., 'Monitoring Nurse–Patient Conversation in a Ward', *Nursing Times*, 30 August 1979, pp. 95–6.

—— 'Nursing as a Research Based Profession', *Nursing Focus*, August 1980, p. 477.

Field, D., *Nursing the Dying*, London: Tavistock/Routledge, 1989.

Field, P., *Attitudes Revisited: An Examination of Student Nurses' Attitudes towards Old People in Hospital*, London: Royal College of Nursing, 1986.

Fineberg, H., 'Screening and Public Health Policy', The Second International Conference on Health Law and Ethics, plenary session paper, 1 July 1989, London.

Flanagan, O. and Jackson, K., 'Justice, Care and Gender: the Kohlberg–Gilligan Debate Revisited', *Ethics*, 1987, vol. 97, pp. 622–37.

Freund, P. A., 'Introduction: Ethical Aspects of Experimentation with Human Subjects', *Daedalus* (Spring 1969), pp. 10–25.

Fry, S. T., 'Toward a Theory of Nursing Ethics', *Advances in Nursing Science*, 1989, vol. 11 (4), pp. 9–22.

Gallagher-Allred, C. R., 'Nutritional Care of the Terminally Ill Patient and Family', in Penson, J. and Fisher, R. (eds), *Palliative Care for People with Cancer*, London : Edward Arnold, 1989, ch. 6, pp. 91–104.

General Medical Council, *Proposals for New Performance Procedures: A Consultation Paper*, London, GMC, May 1992.

Gilligan, C., *In a Different Voice*, Cambridge, Mass.: Harvard University Press, 1982.

Girard, M., 'Technical Expertise as an Ethical Form: Towards an Ethics of Distance', *Journal of Medical Ethics*, 1988, vol. 14, pp. 25–30.

Glaser, B. G. and Strauss, A. L., *Awareness of Dying*, Chicago: Aldine, 1965.

Glazer, M., 'Ten Whistleblowers and how they Fared', *Hastings Center Report*, 1983, vol. 13 (6), pp. 33–41.

Goodey, C. F. (ed.), *Living in the Real World: Families Speak about Down's Syndrome*, London: The Twenty-One Press, 1991.

Gorovitz, S. and Maklin, R., *Moral Problems in Medicine*, Englewood Cliffs: Prentice-Hall, 2nd edn, 1983.

Grant, J. and Hamilton, S., 'Falls in a Rehabilitation Centre: A Retrospective and Comparative Analysis', *Rehabilitation Nursing*, 1987, vol. 12, pp. 74–7.

Green, J. A., 'Minimizing Malpractice Risks by Role Clarification', *Annals of Internal Medicine*, 1 August 1988, pp. 234–6.

Green, R. M., 'Health Care and Justice in Contract Theory Perspective', in Veatch, R. M. and Branson, R. (eds), op. cit., 1976.

Greengross, S. (ed.), *The Law and Vulnerable Elderly People*, Age Concern, London: Mitcham, 1986.

Gunn, M., 'The Law and Mental Handicap: Consent to Treatment', *Mental Handicap*, 1985, vol. 13, pp. 70–2.

Gutheil, T. G., Barsztajn, H. and Brodsky, A., 'Malpractice Prevention through the Sharing of Uncertainty: Informed Consent and the Therapeutic Alliance', *New England Journal of Medicine*, 1984, vol. 311, pp. 49–51.

Habermas, J., *The Theory of Communicative Action*: vol. 2, *The Critique of Functionalist Reason*, Cambridge: Polity, 1987, pp. 113–98.

Hannah, A. I., 'Child Protection. The Way Forward: Some Legal Aspects of the Subject of Child Abuse', Greenwich Health Authority paper, 1989.

Harris, J., *The Value of Life: An Introduction to Medical Ethics*, London: Routledge & Kegan Paul, 1985.

Harvey, G., 'An Evaluation of Approaches to Assessing the Quality of Nursing Care Using (Predetermined) Quality Assurance Tools', *Journal of Advanced Nursing*, 1991, vol. 16, pp. 277–86.

Health and Safety Commission, *Control of Substances Hazardous to Health Regulations*, London: Department of Health, 1989.

Hewa, S. and Hetherington, R. W., 'Specialists without Spirit: Crisis in the Nursing Profession', *Journal of Medical Ethics*, 1990, vol. 16, pp. 179–84.

Heywood Jones, I., *The Nurse's Code*, London: Nursing Times and Macmillan, 1990.

Holden, P. and Littlewood, J. (eds), *Anthropology and Nursing*, London: Routledge, 1991.

Holmes, H. B. and Purdy, L. M. (eds), *Feminist Perspectives in Medical Ethics*, Indiana: Indiana University Press, 1992.

Holmes, P., 'The Patient's Friend', *Nursing Times*, 1991, vol. 87 (19), pp. 16–17.

Hugman, R., *Power in Caring Professions*, London: Macmillan, 1991.

Hunt, G., '"Patient Choice" and the National Health Service Review', *Journal of Social Welfare Law*, 1990, vol. 4, pp. 245–55.

—— 'Nursing, Patient Choice and the NHS Reforms', National Board for Nursing, Midwifery and Health Visiting for Northern Ireland, Occasional Paper, Fourth Annual Celebrity Lecture, Belfast, October 1991.

—— *Nursing Standard*, 'Professional Accountability', 1991, vol. 6 (4), pp. 49–50.

—— *Nursing Standard*, 'Upward Accountability', 1992, vol. 6 (16), pp. 46–7.

—— *Nursing Standard*, 'Downward Accountability', 1992, vol. 6 (21), pp. 44–5.

—— 'Project 2000 – Ethics, Ambivalence and Ideology', in O. Slevin and M. Buckenham (eds), *Project 2000: The Teachers Speak*, Edinburgh: Campion Press, 1992.

—— 'Local Research Ethics Committees and Nursing: A Critical Look', *British Journal of Nursing*, 1992, vol 1. (7), pp. 349–51.

—— 'Changing the Code', *Nursing Times*, 1992, vol. 88 (25), pp. 21–2.

—— 'De verpleegkundige zorg voor chronisch zieken', *Vakblad voor verpleegkundigen*, 1992, vol. 19, pp. 677–82.

Hunt, G. and Wainwright, P. (eds), *Expanding the Role of the Nurse*, Oxford: Blackwell Scientific, 1994.

Illich, I., *Disabling Professions*, London: Marion Boyars, 1987.

Institute of Medical Ethics, 'Medical Confidentiality', *Briefings in Medical Ethics*, 1990, no. 7.

Jirovec, M. M., 'Research with Cognitively Impaired Older Adults: Issues of Informed Consent', *Michigan Nurse*, 1989, vol. 62, pp. 6–15.

Johnson, T. J., *Professions and Power*, London: Macmillan, 1972.

Katz, A., 'Process Design for Selection of Haemodialysis and Organ Transplant Recipients,' *Buffalo Law Review*, 1973, vol. 22, pp. 30–45.

Kennedy, A., 'In the Name of Epidemiology: The Surveillance of HIV and AIDS', unpublished MA thesis, 1989, University of Wales.

Kennedy, I., 'The Legal Effect of Requests by the Terminally Ill and Aged not to Receive Further Treatment from Doctors,' *Criminal Law Review*, April 1976.

Kennedy, I. and Grubb, A., *Medical Law: Text and Materials*, London: Butterworth, 1989.

Kennett, A., 'Informed Consent: A Patient's Right', *The Professional Nurse*, December 1986, pp. 75–7.

Kultgen, J., 'The Ideological Use of Professional Codes', in J. C. Callahan, *Ethical Issues In Professional Life*, New York and Oxford : Oxford University Press, 1988, pp. 411–21; also in *Business and Professional Ethics Journal*, 1982, vol. 1 (3), pp. 53–69.

Lamerton, R., *Care of the Dying*, London: Priory Press, 1973.

Lawler, J., *Behind the Screens: Nursing, Somology, and the Problem of the Body*, Melbourne: Churchill Livingstone, 1991.

Lee, S., 'Judges, Human Rights and the Sources of Medical Law', in P. Byrne (ed.), *Health, Rights and Resources : Kings College Studies 1987–88*, London: King Edward's Hospital Fund for London, 1988, pp. 53–4.

Leenders, F., 'Children First', *Community Outlook*, July 1990, pp. 4–6.

Levine, R. J., *The Ethics and Regulation of Clinical Research*, Baltimore: Urban & Schwarzenberg, 2nd edn, 1986.

Ley, P., 'Psychological Studies of Doctor–Patient Communication', in *Contributions to Medical Psychology*, vol. 1, Oxford: Pergamon, 1977, pp. 9–42.

Lynn, J. and Childress, J. F., 'Must Patients Always be Given Food and Water?' *Hastings Center Report*, 1983, vol. 13 , pp. 17–21.

MacIlwaine, H., 'The Communication Patterns of Female Neurotic Patients with Nursing Staff in Psychiatric Units of General Hospitals', in J. Wilson-Barnett (ed.), *Nursing Research : Ten Studies in Patient Care*, Chichester : John Wiley & Sons, 1983, pp. 1–24.

MacIntyre, A., *After Virtue: A Study in Moral Theory*, London: Duckworth, 2nd edn, 1985.

McKinlay, J., 'On the Professional Regulation of Change', in P. Halmos (ed.), *Professionalisation and Social Change* (Sociological Review Monograph No. 20), Keele: University of Keele Press, 1973.

Macleod Clark, J., 'Nurse–Patient Communication: an Analysis of Conversations from Surgical Wards', in J. Wilson-Barnett (ed.), op. cit., 1983, pp. 25–56.

McLoughlin, J. and Williams, G., 'Alternatives to Prostatectomy', *British Journal of Urology*, 1990, vol. 5, pp. 313–16.

Masters, W. H. and Johnson, V. E., *Human Sexual Response*, London: J. & A. Churchill, 1966.

Medical Research Council, *The Ethical Conduct of Research on the Mentally Incapacitated*, London: MRC, 1991.

—— *Responsibility in Investigations on Human Participants and Materials and on Personal Information*, London: MRC, 1992.

Millard, R., 'The New Accountability', *Nursing Outlook*, 1975, vol. 23 (8), pp. 496–500.

Morrow, G. R., Hoagland, H. C. and Carpenter, E. J., 'Improving Physician–Patient Communications in Cancer Treatment', *Journal of Psychosocial Oncology*, 1983, vol. 1, pp. 93–101.

Muyskens, J. L., *Moral Problems in Nursing: A Philosophical Investigation*, Totowa, N.J.: Rowman & Littlefield, 1982.

—— 'The Nurse as an Employee', in J. C. Callahan (ed.), 1988, op. cit. pp. 110–30.

National Association of Social Workers (NASW) (USA), Code of Conduct, Appendix 1 of the *Encyclopedia of Social Work* (18th edn), ed. Anne Minahan *et al.*, Silver Spring, Md. National Association of Social Workers, 1987.

National Consumer Council, *Patients' Rights: A Guide for N.H.S. Patients and Doctors*, London: NCC, 1983.

National Health Service (NHS) Management Executive, *A Guide to Consent for Examination for Treatment*, London: Department of Health, 1990.

Neuberger, J., *Ethics and Health Care: The Role of Research Ethics Committees in the United Kingdom*, London: King's Fund Institute, 1992.

Noddings, N., *Caring: A Feminine Approach to Ethics and Moral Education*, Berkeley and Los Angeles: University of California Press, 1984.

Noddings, N., 'Do we Really Want to Produce Good People?', *Journal of Moral Education*, 1987, vol. 16 (3), pp. 181–90.

Norberg, A., Asplund, K. and Waxman, H., 'Withdrawing Feeding and Withholding Artificial Nutrition from Severely Demented Patients. Interviews with Care-givers', *Western Journal of Nursing Research*, 1987, vol. 9 (3), pp. 348–56.

Norberg, A., Norberg, B. and Bexell, G., 'Ethical Problems in Feeding Patients with Advanced Dementia', *British Medical Journal*, 1980, vol. 281, pp. 847–8.

Norberg, A., Norberg, B., Gippert, H. and Bexell, G., 'Ethical Conflicts in Long-term Care of the Aged: Nutritional Problems and the Patient–care Worker Relationship', *British Medical Journal*, 1980, vol. 280, pp. 377–8.

Okin, S. M., 'Reason and Feeling in Thinking About Justice', *Ethics*, 1989, vol. 99, pp. 229–49.

Omery, A., 'Moral Development: a Differential Evaluation of Dominant Models', *Advances in Nursing Science*, 1983, vol. 6 (1), pp. 1–17.

Outka, G., 'Social Justice and Equal Access to Health Care', *Journal of Religious Ethics*, vol. 2 (Spring 1974), pp. 11–32.

Owens, P. and Glennerster, H. (eds), *Nursing in Conflict*, London: Macmillan, 1990.

Padfield, C., *Law made Simple*, revised by F.E. Smith, 6th edn, London: Heinemann, 1983.

Parent, W. A., 'Privacy, Morality, and the Law', in J. C. Callahan, *Ethical Issues in Professional Life*, New York and Oxford: Oxford University Press, 1988, pp. 216–36.

Penson, J. and Fisher, R. (eds), *Palliative Care for People with Cancer*, London: Edward Arnold, 1989.

Phillips, M., Commentary on Tony Bland case, *The Guardian*, 5 February 1993.

Printz, L. A., 'Is Withholding Hydration a Valid Comfort Measure?' *Geriatrics*, 1988, vol. 43 (11), pp. 84–8.

Pyne, R., 'Changing the Code', *Nursing Times*, vol. 88 (17 June 1992), pp. 20–1.

—— *Professional Discipline in Nursing, Midwifery and Health Visiting*, Oxford: Blackwell Scientific, 2nd edn, 1992.

Ramsey, P., *The Patient as Person: Explorations in Medical Ethics*, New Haven, Conn.: Yale University Press, 1970.

Redfern, S., 'The Elderly Patient', in Redfern, S. (ed.), *Nursing Elderly People*, Edinburgh: Churchill Livingstone, 2nd edn., 1991, pp. 551–60.

Robinson, J., *A Patient Voice at the GMC: A Lay Member's View of the General Medical Council*, London: Health Rights, 1988.

Royal College of Nursing (RCN), *Accountability in Nursing*, London: RCN, 1980.

—— *Issues in Nursing and Health*, London: RCN, 1992.

Royal College of Physicians (RCP), *Guidelines on the Practice of Ethics Committees in Medical Research Involving Human Subjects*, London: RCP, 1990.

Salvage, J., *The Politics of Nursing*, London: Heinemann, 1985.

Sanders, D. and Dukeminier, J., 'Medical Advance and Legal Lag', *U.C.L.A. Law Review* v. 15, 1968, pp. 377–8.

Savage, J., *Nurses, Gender and Sexuality*, London: Heinemann, 1987.

Savage, W., *A Savage Inquiry: Who Controls Childbirth?*London: Virago, 1986.

Schutz, A. and Luckmann, T., *The Structure of the Lifeworld*, London: Heinemann, 1974.

Scott, G. E., *Moral Personhood*, Albany: State University of New York Press, 1990.

Secord, P. and Backman, C., *Social Psychology*, London: McGraw-Hill, 1964.

Sherlock, R., 'Reasonable Men and Sick Human Beings', *The American Journal of Medicine*, 1986, vol. 80, pp. 2–4.

Simes, R. J., Tottersall, M. H., Coates, A. S. *et al.*, 'A Randomised Comparison of Procedures for Obtaining Informed Consent in Clinical Trials of Treatment for Cancer', *British Medical Journal*, 1986, vol. 293 (6554), pp. 1065–8.

Simon, R., 'Silent Suicide in the Elderly', *Bulletin of the American Academy of Psychiatry*, 1989, vol. 17 (1), pp. 83–95.

Skegg, P. D. G., *Law, Ethics and Medicine*, Oxford: Oxford University Press, 1984.

Smith, L., 'Falls Among the Elderly in an Institutional Setting: Implications for Nurse Education', unpublished M.Sc. thesis, Age Concern Institute of Gerontology, King's College, University of London, London, 1991.

Sterling, E. D. and Yahne, C., 'Surgical Informed Consent: What It Is and What It Is Not', *The American Journal of Surgery*, 1987, vol. 154, pp. 574–8.

Stocks, J. L., *Morality and Purpose*, London: Routledge & Kegan Paul, 1969.

Stockwell, F., *The Unpopular Patient*, London: Royal College of Nursing, 1972.

Thorpe, L., 'Informed Decision-Making', *Nursing*, 1989, vol. 3 (42), pp. 16–19.

Tingle, J. H., 'Negligence and Wilsher', *Solicitors Journal*, 1988, vol. 132 (25), pp. 910–11.

—— 'Medical Paternalism: Blowing the Whistle', *Solicitors Journal*, 1989, vol. 133 (44), p. 3.

—— 'The Important Case of Bull', *Nursing Standard*, 1990, vol. 4 (37), pp. 54–5.

Tomalin, D. A., Redfern, S. J. and Norman, I. J., 'Monitor and Senior Monitor: Problems of Administration and Some Proposed Solutions', *Journal of Advanced Nursing*, 1992, vol. 17, p. 76.

Townsend, P., *Poverty in the United Kingdom: A Survey of Household Resources and Standards of Living*, Harmondsworth: Penguin, 1979.

Treece, E. W. and Treece, J. W., *Elements of Research in Nursing*, St Louis: The C. V. Mosby Company, 1977, pp. 39–40.

Tronto, J. C., 'Beyond Gender Difference to a Theory of Care', *Signs*, 1987, vol. 12 (4), pp. 644–63.

Turner, B. S., *Medical Power and Social Knowledge*, London: Sage, 1987.

Turner, T., 'Crushed by the System', *Nursing Times*, 1990, vol. 86 (49), p. 19.

United Kingdom Central Council for Nursing, Midwifery and Health Visiting (UKCC), *Administration of Medicines*, London: UKCC, 1986.

—— *Confidentiality*, London: UKCC, 1987.

—— *Exercising Accountability*, London: UKCC, 1989.

—— 'with a view to removal from the register...', London: UKCC, 1990.

—— *The Scope of Professional Practice*, London: UKCC, 1992.

—— *The Code of Professional Conduct for the Nurse, Midwife and Health Visitor*, London: UKCC, 3rd edn, June 1992.

—— Annexa (RHP/CS 2) to Registrar's Letter 8/1992, a Council Position Statement on AIDS and HIV Infection (1992).

Veatch, R. M., *Death, Dying and the Biological Revolution: Our Last Quest for Responsibility*, New Haven: Yale University Press, revised edn, 1989.

Veatch, R. M. and Branson, R. (eds), *Ethics and Health Policy*, Cambridge, Mass.: Ballinger Publishing, 1976.

Veatch, R. M. and Fry, S. T., *Case Studies in Nursing Ethics*, Philadelphia: J.B. Lippincott Co., 1987.

Wainwright, P. J., 'Qualpacs - a Practical Guide', in *The Ward Sister's Survival Guide*, London: Austen Cornish Publishers Ltd, 1990, pp.171-5.

Wandelt, M. and Ager, J., *Quality Patient Care Scale*, New York: Appleton Century Crofts, 1974.

Warnock, M., 'A National Ethics Committee', *British Medical Journal*, 1988, vol. 297, pp. 1626-7.

Waterworth, S. and Luker, K. A., 'Reluctant Collaborations: Do Patients Want to be Involved in Decisions Concerning Care?' *Journal of Advanced Nursing*, 1990, vol. 15, pp. 971-6.

Watts, D. T. and Cassel, C. K., 'Extraordinary Nutritional Support: A Case Study and Ethical Analysis', *Journal of the American Geriatrics Society*, 1984, vol. 32 (3), pp. 237-42.

Wells, W. T., 'Medicine and the Law: The Surgeon's Duty to Warn of Risk', *The Lancet*, 28 April 1984, p. 974.

Wieder, D. L., 'Telling the Code', in R. Turner (ed.), *Ethnomethodology*, Harmondsworth: Penguin, 1974, pp. 161-2.

Wiles, A., 'Quality of Patient Care Scale', in A. Pearson (ed.), *Nursing Quality Measurement*, Chichester: John Wiley & Sons, p. 29.

Wilson-Barnett, J. (ed.), *Nursing Research: Ten Studies in Patient Care*, Chichester: John Wiley & Sons, 1983.

Winston, K. M. and Mebust, M. D., 'Surgical Management of Benign Prostatic Obstruction', *Supplement to Urology*, 1988, vol. 32, pp. 574-77.

World Health Organisation, *International Classification of Impairments, Disabilities and Handicap*, Geneva: WHO, 1980.

Young, A., *Legal Problems in Nursing Practice*, London: Chapman and Hall, 2nd edn, 1989.

—— *Law and Professional Conduct in Nursing*, London: Scutari, 1991.

Zerwekh, J. V., 'The Dehydration Question', *Nursing*, 1983, vol. 83 (13), pp. 47-51.

Index